Current Practices in Ophthalmology

Series Editor

Parul Ichhpujani
Department of Ophthalmology
Government Medical College and Hospital
Chandigarh, India

This series of highly organized and uniform handbooks aims to cover the latest clinically relevant developments in ophthalmology. In the wake of rapidly evolving innovations in the field of basic research, pharmacology, surgical techniques and imaging devices for the management of ophthalmic disorders, it is extremely important to invest in books that help you stay updated. These handbooks are designed to bridge the gap between journals and standard texts providing reviews on advances that are now part of mainstream clinical practice. Meant for residents, fellows-in-training, generalist ophthalmologists and specialists alike, each volume under this series covers current perspectives on relevant topics and meets the CME requirements as a go-to reference guide. Supervised and reviewed by a subject expert, chapters in each volume provide leading-edge information most relevant and useful for clinical ophthalmologists. This series is also useful for residents and fellows training in various subspecialties of ophthalmology, who can read these books while at work or during emergency duties. Additionally, these handbooks can aid in preparing for clinical case discussions at various forums and examinations.

More information about this series at http://www.springer.com/series/15743

Aparna Ramasubramanian

Editor

Ocular Oncology

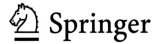 Springer

Editor
Aparna Ramasubramanian
University of Louisville
Louisville, KY
USA

ISSN 2523-3807   ISSN 2523-3815   (electronic)
Current Practices in Ophthalmology
ISBN 978-981-13-7537-8   ISBN 978-981-13-7538-5   (eBook)
https://doi.org/10.1007/978-981-13-7538-5

This Springer imprint is published by the registered company Springer Nature Singapore Pte Ltd.
The registered company address is: 152 Beach Road, #21-01/04 Gateway East, Singapore 189721, Singapore

Contents

About the Editor

Aparna Ramasubramanian is an assistant professor of pediatric ophthalmology and oncology at the University of Louisville. She did her medical school at the University of Kerala, India, followed by ophthalmology residency in Indiana University. She received fellowship training in ocular oncology at Wills Eye Institute and in pediatric ophthalmology at Children's Hospital, Boston. Her primary research and clinical interest is retinoblastoma, and she is the author of the leading textbook on *Retinoblastoma*. She has published extensively in peer-reviewed journals and is a reviewer for all leading ophthalmology journals. Besides retinoblastoma, she also treats the whole range of pediatric and adult eye tumors and keeps a keen interest in secondary eye manifestations of cancer.

Current Management in Retinoblastoma

Shweta Gupta and Swathi Kaliki

Introduction

Management of retinoblastoma is complex as well as highly customized for every single child. The choice of treatment depends on many factors including age of the patient at presentation, tumor laterality, tumor size and location, macular involvement, vitreous and/or subretinal seeding, tumor relationship to surrounding tissues (optic disc, choroid, iris, sclera, and orbit), tumor staging, risk for metastasis, and visual potential [1, 2]. It involves certain considerations such as systemic status, overall prognosis as well as family desires, social perception, and cost-effectiveness of treatment in a particular financial setting.

The principal objective of retinoblastoma treatment is child survival, followed by globe salvage and preservation of vision. It is a challenge to cure the disease and preserve the globe while maximizing visual potential and minimizing toxicity. A multidisciplinary approach at a tertiary care center is fundamental in the treatment of retinoblastoma with an organized team comprising ocular oncologist, pediatric oncologist, ocular pathologist, pediatrician, interventional radiologist, radiotherapist, and genetic counselor [3]. It involves grouping and staging of tumor, decision about the appropriate treatment modality, careful follow-up for assessment of treatment response, and early detection of recurrence. International Classification for Intraocular Retinoblastoma is currently used for the grouping of intraocular retinoblastoma [4]. It helps to predict the treatment success as well as high-risk disease on histopathology [5, 6]. Staging of the tumor is done according to International Retinoblastoma Staging System (IRSS) [7]. The recommended initial metastatic workup includes lumbar puncture for cerebrospinal fluid analysis (CSF),

S. Gupta · S. Kaliki (✉)
The Operation Eyesight Universal Institute for Eye Cancer, L V Prasad Eye Institute, Hyderabad, Telangana, India

© Springer Nature Singapore Pte Ltd. 2019
A. Ramasubramanian (ed.), *Ocular Oncology*, Current Practices in Ophthalmology, https://doi.org/10.1007/978-981-13-7538-5_1

bone marrow biopsy, and bone scan. It is suggested that these tests are essential in stage III and IV patients to rule out micrometastasis and stage II patients need further evaluation but there is no role of these investigations in stage 0 and I retinoblastoma [8].

Various modalities in the treatment of retinoblastoma can be classified into focal therapy (transpupillary thermotherapy, laser photocoagulation, cryotherapy, plaque brachytherapy), local therapy (intra-arterial chemotherapy, enucleation, external beam radiotherapy/EBRT), and systemic therapy (intravenous chemotherapy). Small tumors are primarily treated with focal therapy, while local and systemic modalities are used in the treatment of advanced retinoblastoma [9]. There are several management options for children with unilateral sporadic intraocular retinoblastoma depending on the tumor group based on the International Classification for Intraocular Retinoblastoma (ICIOR) [4]. Traditionally, small-size tumors with minimal subretinal fluid are controlled with transpupillary thermotherapy or cryotherapy. Tumors with large size and more extensive subretinal fluid or seeding receive chemoreduction along with consolidation measures. Majority of children with bilateral retinoblastoma are treated with intravenous chemoreduction and patients with orbital retinoblastoma undergo orbital exenteration [3].

There has been remarkable advancement in the conservative treatment of intraocular as well as orbital retinoblastoma over the last decade, using different routes of drug delivery, new chemotherapeutic agents, and novel radiation treatment modalities in order to improve success rates and minimize the adverse effects of conventional treatment.

Conservative treatment modalities which salvage the globe as well as preserve functional vision are increasingly being used for less advanced disease (groups A–D ICIOR) [10]. These include systemic chemotherapy, intra-arterial chemotherapy, focal consolidation, radiation treatment with plaque brachytherapy, and local injections of chemotherapeutic agents through the intravitreal/subtenon's route in addition to systemic chemotherapy.

Chemotherapy

Role of chemotherapy in the management of retinoblastoma is gradually increasing with the introduction of newer globe salvage strategies. Although innovative delivery routes are being initiated, intravenous chemotherapy remains the most widely used treatment modality. New targeted therapies deliver the drug directly to the tumor with reduced side effects to the adjoining normal retina as well as systemic health.

Intravenous Chemotherapy

A triple-drug therapy with vincristine, etoposide, and carboplatin (VEC) is most commonly used for intravenous chemotherapy and remains standard first-line conservative therapy worldwide (Fig. 1).

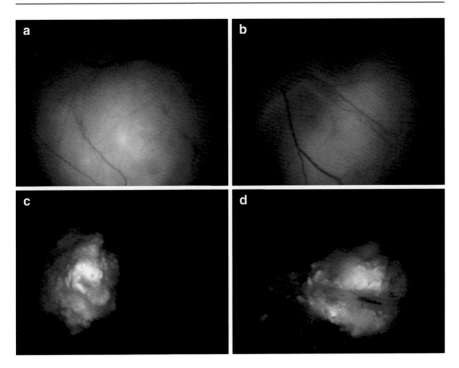

Fig. 1 Intravenous chemotherapy for retinoblastoma. A child with bilateral retinoblastoma with total retinal detachment (**a, b**) responded well with six cycles of chemotherapy with type 1 regression (**c, d**) of tumors in both eyes

The various indications of systemic chemotherapy in management of retinoblastoma can be described as

- Chemoreduction for primary intraocular retinoblastoma (especially large group B–D tumors)
- Chemoprophylaxis/adjuvant chemotherapy for post-enucleation patients with high-risk histopathological features
- Orbital retinoblastoma (neoadjuvant and adjuvant therapy)
- Palliative treatment for metastatic retinoblastoma
- Salvage treatment for recurrent or refractory tumor

Intravenous chemotherapy can be used in primary management of all retinoblastoma tumors. Standard dose (SD) of the three-drug combination is commonly used in majority of cases [11]. High-dose (HD) chemotherapy is advised in advanced cases and tumors unresponsive to standard dose chemotherapy [9] (Table 1). Treatment is generally given 3–4 weekly up to six cycles and tumor response is assessed at examination under anesthesia prior to each cycle of chemotherapy.

Treatment success with chemotherapy alone has been observed in 100%, 93%, and 90% of ICIOR group A, B, and C eyes, respectively [3, 5, 12]. Success rates for

Table 1 Chemotherapy drugs, dose, and treatment schedule for retinoblastoma

Drug	Standard dose (<3 years of age)	Standard dose (>3 years of age)	High dose
Vincristine	0.05 mg/kg	1.5 mg/m^2	0.025 mg/kg
Etoposide	5 mg/kg	150 mg/m^2	12 mg/kg
Carboplatin	18.6 mg/kg	560 mg/m^2	28 mg/kg

Day 1: Vincristine + etoposide + carboplatin
Day 2: Etoposide

globe salvage decrease with advancing intraocular grade. Suboptimal tumor regression is seen in ICIOR group D and E eyes and approximately half of the eyes in group D require EBRT or enucleation for tumor control [5]. With increasing use of intravitreal chemotherapy, the globe salvage rates of group D eyes have increased and the need for EBRT has decreased. Systemic chemotherapy is often combined with local therapy as it reduces the size and volume of the tumor as well as makes them responsive to local therapy [11, 13–15]. Some (18–62%) eyes show tumor recurrence in the form of vitreous seeds and subretinal seeds with the six-cycle regimen of VEC and can be salvaged with thermotherapy, cryotherapy, or plaque radiotherapy [16, 17].

Intravenous chemotherapy covers both eyes simultaneously, and prevents pinealoblastoma, secondary cancers, and systemic metastasis [3, 18]. Chemoreduction still remains a vital treatment option for patients with bilateral retinoblastoma or those with advanced disease as initial therapy [3]. Extensive retinoblastoma in group E eyes is most difficult to treat, which is generally managed with enucleation. However, with chemoreduction an attempt to save at least one eye can be made in cases with bilateral group E retinoblastoma [19]. Group E eyes treated with chemoreduction and low-dose (2600 cGy) prophylactic radiotherapy showed significantly fewer recurrences than those treated with chemoreduction alone. Globe salvage rate of 22–70% was noticed with combination of chemotherapy and radiation in eyes with vitreous seeds [20].

Treatment of retinoblastoma involves thorough interpretation of tumor regression, tumor activity, and early identification of recurrence. There are five types of regression patterns described in retinoblastoma including type 0 (no scar), type 1 (calcified), type 2 (noncalcified), type 3 (partially calcified), and type 4 (flat scar). Smaller tumors commonly regress to types 0, 2, and 4, whereas larger tumors to type 1 or 3 [3]. Careful follow-up of treated patients is recommended because of significant risk for recurrent vitreous and subretinal seeds followed by appropriate treatment of the recurrent lesion for complete tumor control [11].

Before commencing the intravenous chemotherapy, it is necessary to ensure the blood counts such as absolute neutrophil count >1000/mm^3 and platelets >1 lac/mm^3. Acute toxicity expected with systemic chemotherapy includes pancytopenia resulting in anemia, thrombocytopenia and neutropenia, alopecia, fever, and weight loss. Long-term side effects of the chemotherapy are renal dysfunction, high-frequency hearing loss, peripheral neuropathy, and second malignancy including leukemia. Although uncommon, screening for these potential late effects should be integrated in the follow-up [21].

Intra-arterial Chemotherapy (IAC)

New treatment approaches with localized delivery of chemotherapy minimize the systemic side effects of intravenous chemotherapy. Intra-arterial chemotherapy is one such novel approach, which delivers chemotherapy directly to the eye with the tumor through the ophthalmic artery and has fewer systemic side effects [22]. There has been evolution in the technique from selective ophthalmic artery infusion, where a microballoon catheter was positioned by a transfemoral artery approach at the cervical segment of the internal carotid artery just distal to the orifice of the ophthalmic artery to technique of super-selective intra-arterial infusion by advancing a microcatheter directly into the orifice of the ophthalmic artery [22–24]. Melphalan (5 mg, 7.5 mg) is the drug of choice for intra-arterial chemotherapy, topotecan (1 mg) is additional in cases with extensive vitreous seeding, while three-drug regimen including carboplatin is administered in advanced cases. Treatment is repeated every 4 weeks and majority of patients require three chemotherapy sessions for complete tumor control.

Intra-arterial chemotherapy is emerging as a safe and effective treatment modality for advanced intraocular retinoblastoma. It can be used either as a primary treatment, particularly in unilateral cases to avoid systemic therapy and enucleation or as secondary treatment in recalcitrant and recurrent retinoblastoma (Fig. 2). Shields

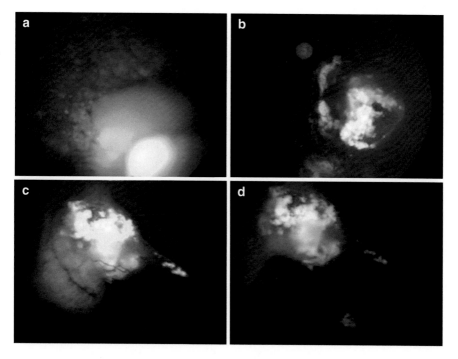

Fig. 2 Intra-arterial chemotherapy for retinoblastoma. (**a**) A 4-year-old child with failed systemic chemotherapy with massive tumor recurrence with diffuse subretinal and vitreous seeds responded well (**b**) with four cycles of intra-arterial chemotherapy. (**c**) A 3-year-old child with failed systemic chemotherapy with massive tumor recurrence responded well (**d**) with two cycles of intra-arterial chemotherapy

et al. noted globe salvage in 94% group D eyes and vitreous seed regression in 91% eyes with IAC used as primary therapy. There was superior globe salvage in group D eyes as well as better control for solid tumor, subretinal seeds, and vitreous seeds in comparison to intravenous chemotherapy [25, 26]. In 96% of group D treatment-naive eyes, complete regression of the main tumor was achieved with three sessions of intra-arterial chemotherapy in majority of cases. Tuncer et al. concluded that management of advanced intraocular retinoblastoma primarily with intra-arterial chemotherapy could avoid enucleation or external beam radiotherapy in most of the eyes [27]. Shields et al. found that IAC with additional intravitreal chemotherapy for vitreous seeding improved globe salvage in eyes with advanced untreated unilateral retinoblastoma [28]. IAC can be an effective second- or third-line therapy in the management of massive persistent or recurrent subretinal seeds following previous chemotherapy [29]. Successful salvage of 50% of eyes has been reported in recurrent and refractory retinoblastoma [22, 30, 31]. Primary intravenous chemotherapy followed by secondary IAC provides globe salvage in 57% of the eyes with advanced retinoblastoma (groups D and E) [32]. Eyes with vitreous seeds require higher treatment sessions and multiple drugs compared to eyes without vitreous seeds. IAC has been shown to be more effective in eyes with vitreous seeds that had previous treatment failure in comparison to previously treated eyes with subretinal seeds [33].

Intra-arterial chemotherapy is mostly preferred in unilateral nongermline mutation retinoblastoma. However, simultaneous bilateral intra-arterial chemotherapy for bilateral retinoblastoma has also been reported with globe salvage in 95% of eyes [34]. IAC can also be considered as a rescue therapy using melphalan alone or with additional topotecan in children with recurrent retinoblastoma in the only eye (especially if the opposite eye had been enucleated) with previous IAC failure. It provided tumor control in 75% of cases and globe salvage in 67% [35]. Three sessions of intra-arterial topotecan–melphalan chemotherapy are effective for preventing enucleation in 55% of affected eyes in single-eyed children [36]. IAC has shown encouraging results in the treatment of retinoblastoma in infants <3 months of age as primary therapy [37]. Tumor regression can also be achieved in adult-onset recurrent retinoblastoma [38].

Local side effects of IAC include transient ipsilateral eyelid edema, blepharoptosis, forehead hyperemia, third cranial nerve palsy, orbital edema, diffuse choroidal atrophy, retinal detachment, vitreous hemorrhage, and transient pancytopenia. However, no cases of hematologic toxicity or cerebrovascular accident from this technique have been reported till date [39, 40]. Another serious concern with IAC is embolic events to the globe, which range from transient ischemia to ophthalmic artery obstruction [26]. Myelosuppression occurs more commonly after triple-agent IAC than single-agent melphalan [41]. It was observed that IAC does not increase the risk of orbital recurrence, metastatic disease, or death compared with primary enucleation when used for advanced intraocular retinoblastoma [42, 43]. The issue regarding difficulty in visualization and catheterization of ophthalmic artery could be dealt with the strategies as illustrated by Bertelli et al. [44].

The technique of IAC has replaced first-line systemic chemotherapy in many countries and is advised as the primary treatment strategy in conservative management of retinoblastoma. However, the concerns regarding the cost and the risk of metastasis still remain at few centers, which makes this approach controversial, and IAC is reserved for second-line treatment of relapsed or refractory disease.

Intravitreal Chemotherapy

Vitreous seeds are collections of tumor cells in the avascular vitreous that are relatively resistant to the intravenous chemotherapy due to lack of blood supply. Vitreous relapse is the biggest challenge in the management of retinoblastoma due to inadequate penetration and suboptimal levels of chemotherapy into the vitreous from intravenous and even intra-arterial routes [16]. Injection of drugs directly into the vitreous overcomes this obstacle, attains better intraocular drug concentration in the vitreous, and efficiently causes regression of vitreous seeds.

Intravitreal chemotherapy is used as a salvage treatment in cases of refractory persistent and recurrent vitreous seeds and is not a primary treatment modality [45]. Intravitreal melphalan is the most effective drug against retinoblastoma and is most widely used for control of vitreous disease [46]. Munier et al. described melphalan as the drug of choice in a dose of 20–30 µg/0.1 mL and discussed a safe technique for intravitreal injection to prevent extraocular extension of the tumor. Any tumor, subretinal fluid, or vitreous seeds at the injection site should be ruled out after meticulous intraocular examination. The drug should be delivered using 29G or 30G needle via pars plana route 3–3.5 mm away from limbus followed by triple-freeze-thaw cryotherapy application at the injection site to avoid escape of tumor cells via the needle track and rotation of globe after taking out the needle for the uniform distribution of drug (Fig. 3). Repeat injection can be given every 7–10 days until regression of the tumor [47–49].

Intravitreal chemotherapy has shown encouraging success in previously treated eyes with vitreous seeding (Fig. 4) [23, 47]. Vitreous seed regression rate of 85–100% and globe salvage rate of 51–100% have been reported in eyes that had already been previously treated with systemic intravenous chemotherapy [23, 49–53]. It is critical to distinguish active vitreous seeding from inactive calcified seeding. The active retinal source of seeding must be identified and treated with focal treatment alone or combined with intra-arterial/intravitreal chemotherapy [49]. Francis et al. evaluated the regression and response of three types of vitreous seeds, i.e., dust, spheres, and clouds, to intravitreal melphalan. Eyes with dust required minimum time to regression with fewer injections while eyes with clouds needed significantly higher cumulative dose of melphalan with greater time for regression [51].

Intravitreal injection is contraindicated in anterior segment or ciliary body invasion, group E retinoblastoma, diffuse vitreous seeds in all quadrants, presence of complete PVD, and total retinal detachment [47, 48]. The reports about effects of

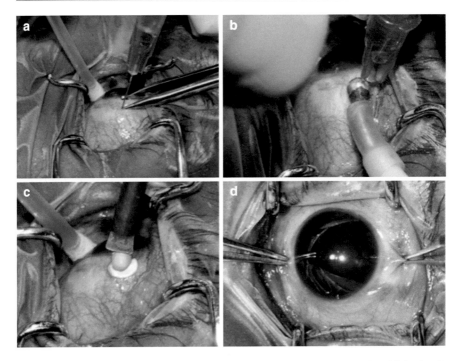

Fig. 3 Technique of intravitreal chemotherapy for retinoblastoma. (**a**) Intravitreal injection is given through pars plana route away from the quadrant of vitreous seeds. (**b**) Postinjection, the needle is withdrawn through the freeze at the injection site. (**c**) Double-freeze-thaw cryotherapy is completed at the injection site. (**d**) The globe is wiggled to allow dispersion of the drug in vitreous

intravitreal chemotherapy on retinal function as studied on electroretinogram are contradictory, which varies from preservation of retinal function to permanent retinal toxicity [54, 55]. The risk of extraocular spread following intravitreal injection in retinoblastoma is negligible when performed using proper technique [23, 53, 56].

Melphalan is not a stable drug and needs to be used within an hour of reconstitution. On the other hand, topotecan has a longer half-life. It is used in a concentration of 8–20 µg/0.04 mL. Combination of intravitreal melphalan (40 µg in 0.04 mL) and topotecan (8–20 µg in 0.04 mL) is found to be safe and effective in cases of extensive vitreous seeding [57].

Periocular/Subtenon's Chemotherapy

Periocular chemotherapy is preferred in advanced group D and E retinoblastoma with diffuse vitreous seeds [58] in the remaining eye of patients with bilateral poor prognosis retinoblastoma where other eye is already enucleated and patients in whom systemic chemotherapy is contraindicated [59]. Periocular injection results

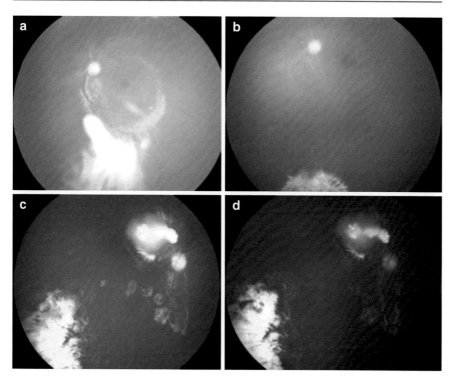

Fig. 4 Intravitreal chemotherapy for retinoblastoma. (**a**) A 2-year-old child with recurrent vitreous seeds responded well (**b**) to six cycles of intravitreal melphalan. (**c**) A 3-year-old child with recurrent vitreous seeds responded well (**d**) to two cycles of intravitreal melphalan

in rapid and augmented vitreous concentration of the drug due to trans-scleral penetration from subtenon's space. Carboplatin (20 mg) or topotecan (1 mg) is dispensed by injection in posterior subtenon's space in the quadrant closest to the location of vitreous seeds. As a single therapy, subtenon's carboplatin showed initial satisfactory results but revealed high failure rate on longer follow-up [60]. Subtenon's chemotherapy improves tumor control when used in combination with intravenous chemoreduction. Group C and D retinoblastoma managed with additional subtenon's carboplatin (20 mg) showed improved tumor control [5, 61]. High-dose intravenous chemotherapy with concurrent periocular carboplatin as a primary treatment modality has shown 95% salvage rate in eyes with focal vitreous seeds and 70% salvage rate in eyes with diffuse vitreous seeds [62]. Single injection of nanoparticle carboplatin has displayed better penetration of chemotherapy in different studies [63, 64]. Side effects of this modality have been described as eyelid edema and ecchymosis, localized subconjunctival hemorrhage, loss of limbal stem cells with conjunctival overgrowth, orbital fat atrophy, muscle fibrosis, optic neuropathy, and orbital cellulitis [59, 61, 65, 66]. Most serious complication of periocular chemotherapy is periorbital scarring, which increases the risk of globe rupture and tumor dissemination in the subsequent enucleation [59]. Recently developed fibrin sealant has shown to deliver sustained and localized concentrations of drug, which would improve the efficacy as well as avoid most of the associated complications [67].

Focal Therapy

Small tumors (group A) away from visually significant areas can be managed with focal treatments alone. Systemic chemotherapy combined with focal therapy remains the standard of care for effective tumor control and globe preservation in early disease (group B–D tumors) [68]. In these cases, focal therapy can be started simultaneously with systemic chemotherapy or is delivered after initial chemoreduction in cases with poor tumor visibility on preliminary examination. Focal treatment modalities help in consolidation after adequate reduction in tumor thickness and resolution in subretinal fluid with chemoreduction. Maximal tumor shrinkage is generally appreciated after the first cycle of chemotherapy and subsequently local therapy can be applied prior to each cycle. Small recurrent tumors arising from subretinal seeds can also be treated with focal treatment.

Cryotherapy

It is indicated in peripheral and equatorial tumors <3.5 mm diameter and <2 mm in thickness. Trans-scleral cryotherapy involves freezing of tumor under visualization using indirect ophthalmoscopy. Triple-freeze-thaw cycles of cryotherapy are applied at 3–4-week interval. Cryotherapy destroys tumor cells mechanically by disruption of cell membranes during thawing of intracellular crystals. It is a critical treatment modality for recurrent subretinal seeds near the ora serrata but it fails in the presence of vitreous seeds overlying the tumor [61]. Main disadvantage of cryotherapy is that it leads to large area of retinal scarring [69].

Transpupillary Thermotherapy (TTT)

It is indicated in posterior tumors <3 mm thickness and <3 mm basal diameter. Fovea-sparing thermotherapy can be used in tumors involving macula or optic disc as it causes lesser visual loss in comparison to laser photocoagulation or radiation. Infrared radiation from semiconductor diode laser (810 nm) generates a slow and sustained temperature (40–60 °C) within the tumor, which subsequently turns the tumor grey and destroys it without affecting the tumor vessels. 1500 μm large spots at a longer duration of 900 ms and 300–540 mW power are dispensed with indirect ophthalmoscope delivery system. It is usually performed along with the intravenous chemoreduction as heat has a synergist effect with chemotherapy [61]. Complete tumor regression has been observed after 3–4 sessions in 85% of cases. Few side effects reported with intense treatment in larger tumors are focal iris atrophy, focal paradoxical lens opacity, retinal traction, and serous retinal detachment [70].

Laser Photocoagulation

It is indicated in posterior tumors with <3 mm diameter and <2 mm thickness not involving macula or optic disc. Argon green laser (532 nm) incorporated in indirect laser delivery system is used for vascular photocoagulation. Confluent spots at 250–350 mW power for 0.3–0.5 s are placed surrounding the tumor base in two rows. Thus restriction of the blood supply to the tumor as well as hyperthermia destroys tumor cells. Direct treatment of tumor is avoided as it could lead to vitreous seeding [61]. Treatment is repeated at 3–4 weeks for three sessions. The side effects are retinal vascular occlusion, retinal hole, retinal scarring, retinal traction, and serous retinal detachment. It is seldom used in view of narrow therapeutic window. It restricts blood supply to the active tumor in patients with ongoing chemotherapy and lowers the concentration of drug inside the tumor. Therefore it is avoided in eyes receiving chemoreduction [1, 71].

There is a debate regarding treatment of macular tumors with focal treatment modalities. They can be observed while on chemotherapy or careful treatment with foveal sparing thermotherapy can be considered to protect the papillomacular bundle. Higher recurrence rates were noticed in those observed without consolidation compared to those consolidated but the majority of recurrent tumors were treated with plaque radiotherapy, thus preserving the vision [72–74].

Radiotherapy

Retinoblastoma is a highly radiosensitive tumor and therefore radiation therapy has an established role in selected patients. It may be in the form of plaque brachytherapy or EBRT.

Episcleral Plaque Brachytherapy

Episcleral plaque radiotherapy is an effective treatment for retinoblastoma (Fig. 5). The plaque, most commonly ruthenium-106 or iodine-125, is placed on the sclera at the base of the tumor and removed after a predetermined duration. The radiation dose and duration of plaque therapy are calculated by dosimetry to provide up to 40 Gy to the tumor apex. It delivers a high dose of radiation to a defined area of the globe while minimizing exposure to surrounding ocular structures.

Special plaques with a notch are used to treat tumors adjacent to the optic disc. It has deeper penetration, simultaneously treats overlying focal vitreous seeds, and commonly requires single treatment session; however it is not ideal for large and

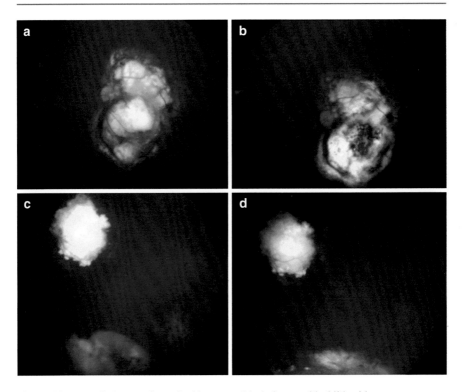

Fig. 5 Plaque radiotherapy for retinoblastoma. (**a**) A 2-year-old child with recurrent tumor responded well (**b**) to plaque radiotherapy. (**c**) A 3-year-old child with persistent subretinal seeds responded well (**d**) to plaque radiotherapy

multifocal recurrent tumors. Side effects of radiation therapy include dry eyes, irritation, madarosis, cataract, scleral necrosis, radiation retinopathy or papillopathy, optic neuropathy, and strabismus. Second malignancies do not appear to be associated with this type of local therapy [61].

Shields et al. reported that plaque radiotherapy provided tumor control in 79% cases with recalcitrant retinoblastoma at 5-year follow-up and best long-term control was observed in tumors without vitreous or subretinal seeding in young patients [75]. Plaque brachytherapy has evolved not only as a secondary treatment modality for recurrent or residual tumor after chemotherapy, focal consolidation, or failed EBRT, but also as a primary treatment [75–77]. Solitary tumors with >3 mm thicknesses that are located anterior to the equator and are not suitable for other forms of focal therapy are amenable to treatment with plaque brachytherapy [78–80]. The American Brachytherapy Society Ophthalmic Oncology Task Force recommends primary brachytherapy for unilateral anterior lesions that are <15 mm in base, <10 mm in thickness, and without vitreous seeding [81]. Tumor control was seen in 88% eyes treated with plaque as primary treatment, in 92% eyes following previously failed chemoreduction, and poorer (75%) in previously failed EBRT with good visual outcomes [79, 80].

External Beam Radiotherapy

External beam radiotherapy was the mainstay of conservative treatment for intraocular retinoblastoma for many decades in the pre-chemotherapy era. At present, the main indications of EBRT are chemoresistant cases of intraocular retinoblastoma (especially multifocal tumor with diffuse vitreous seeds), as an adjuvant therapy in residual microscopic disease after enucleation, and as part of multimodal therapy for orbital retinoblastoma and metastatic disease. It is usually reserved as last treatment alternative for salvage in cases of recalcitrant tumor or vitreous seeds in the only eye with residual vision, where it achieves excellent long-term tumor control. Shields and co-workers commented that group E eyes treated with chemoreduction and low-dose (2600 cGy) prophylactic radiotherapy showed significantly fewer recurrences than those treated with chemoreduction alone [19]. In spite of its proven efficacy, it is no longer a primary globe salvage modality due to considerable risk of late-onset second malignancies in patients with germline mutation and radiation-induced complications such as orbital hypoplasia, dry eye, cataract, and retinopathy.

Radiotherapy is usually delivered as lens-sparing technique using a photon beam. Standard dose is 40–45 Gy, which is generally given in fractions over 3–4 weeks. In recent times, there has been extensive advancement in radiation therapy with the introduction of newer radiotherapy techniques. These include intensity-modulated radiotherapy, stereotactic conformal radiotherapy (SCR), volumetric modulated arc therapy, proton therapy, and helical tomotherapy [82]. SCR is a noninvasive radiotherapy technique that delivers treatment with small beams using highly accurate positioning and can provide an alternative to brachytherapy. It provides more homogeneous dose within the target and lower doses to the surrounding normal tissues [83]. However, additional studies with long-term results are needed to prove its efficacy over plaque therapy. Proton beam therapy provides uniform dose coverage of the target, has no exit dose, and distributes no energy beyond the target like photon beams [84]. It is anticipated that these unique properties of proton beam radiotherapy using linear accelerator may reduce the exposure of normal tissue to the carcinogenic effects of radiation and thus reduce the risk of second cancers in patients with genetic retinoblastoma [21]. However, proton therapy is expensive and is currently not widely available.

Surgery

Enucleation

Enucleation is an effective treatment for retinoblastoma that can be considered as a primary treatment modality or secondary treatment measure in cases of recalcitrant disease after the failure of primary salvage therapy and for orbital retinoblastoma after neoadjuvant chemotherapy. Primary enucleation has been a preferred approach for extensive retinoblastoma specifically if it is unilateral group E and certain unilateral group D eyes with clinical features predictive of high-risk features on histopathology. Kaliki et al. concluded that globe-preserving methods should be used cautiously in patients with secondary glaucoma at presentation and prolonged duration of symptoms (>6 months) [85]. Enucleation is preferred in massive retinoblastoma with no expectation for functional vision [3]. Despite the advances in the salvage treatment modalities, primary enucleation is considered for advanced unilateral cases such as eyes with tumor touching the lens, buphthalmos, pseudohypopyon, hyphema, iris nodules, iris neovascularization, ectropion uveae, dense vitreous hemorrhage, phthisis bulbi, staphyloma, and orbital cellulitis.

It involves careful removal of the globe along with a long section of optic nerve while avoiding globe trauma and tumor seeding into the orbit. Meticulous replacement of the orbital volume with a silicone/PMMA implant by myoconjunctival technique is a safe and cost-effective procedure and provides excellent cosmesis and prosthesis motility [1]. A temporary conformer is placed at the time of surgery, which then later is replaced by a customized prosthesis. Porous implants are avoided in patients with need for adjuvant chemotherapy or EBRT since it may impede the fibrovascular integration of these implants [21].

Post-enucleation histopathological evaluation of globe is crucial to rule out high-risk features. Such cases pose a high risk for local recurrence as well as systemic metastasis and require further chemotherapy and/or radiotherapy [86–89]. Various high-risk features are massive choroidal invasion (>3 mm), retrolaminar optic nerve invasion, optic nerve invasion at transection, scleral and orbital invasion, anterior chamber seeds, iris infiltration, ciliary body infiltration, and combination of prelaminar/laminar optic nerve invasion with any thickness of choroidal infiltration [90–92]. High-risk features were found in 18% of the globes enucleated with retinoblastoma including retrolaminar optic nerve invasion in 10% and massive uveal invasion in 8% [90]. It has been shown that metastasis occurred in 24% of high-risk patients if not treated with adjuvant chemotherapy, whereas only in 4% when treated with adjuvant chemotherapy [92]. At present, all patients with high-risk histopathological features receive 4-weekly six cycles of vincristine, etoposide, and carboplatin [3, 92, 93]. Additionally, presence of tumor cells at the cut end of the optic nerve [21] and full-thickness scleral extension/extra-scleral extension indicates residual microscopic disease and needs intensive chemotherapy as well as orbital radiotherapy [9].

Orbital Exenteration

It is indicated in primary/recurrent orbital tumor that fails to respond to neoadjuvant chemotherapy.

Orbital Retinoblastoma

It is mostly seen in developing countries of Asia and Africa, where extraocular disease constitutes 0.5–50% of all retinoblastoma cases [94–98]. The management of orbital retinoblastoma remains a challenge as orbital involvement is associated with a 10–27 times higher risk of systemic metastasis when compared with cases without orbital extension [99]. However, an effective tumor control can be achieved with thorough systemic workup, intensive multimodal treatment, and careful monitoring. All patients of orbital retinoblastoma undergo baseline computed tomography/magnetic resonance imaging to assess the tumor extent followed by systemic evaluation of metastasis and staging by detailed physical examination, regional lymph node palpation, chest X-ray, ultrasonography of abdomen, bone marrow biopsy, and cerebrospinal fluid cytology [96]. Technetium-99 bone scan or positron emission tomography together with computed tomography could be useful modalities for the early detection of subclinical systemic metastasis [100, 101].

Nowadays, the preferred management approach involves a multimodal protocol, which consists of neoadjuvant high-dose chemotherapy (3–6 cycles) followed by surgery (enucleation/exenteration), EBRT (45–50 Gy), and adjuvant high-dose chemotherapy (6–9 cycles) to complete total 12 cycles [9, 102–104]. Initially, a combination of high-dose chemotherapeutic agents is used to induce tumor regression and to prevent systemic metastasis. Subsequently, surgery and radiotherapy followed by adjuvant high-dose chemotherapy are given till 12 cycles to eradicate microscopic residual disease, and to prevent orbital recurrence and metastasis [96]. It has been suggested to follow up the patient with imaging at 12, 18, 28, and 36 months and bone marrow biopsy and cerebrospinal fluid cytology at 6, 12, 18, 24, and 36 months, respectively, to rule out recurrence and metastasis [96].

Surgery reduces the tumor load and the choice of surgical intervention depends on the etiology of the orbital retinoblastoma in addition to tumor response to neoadjuvant chemotherapy [96, 98]. In primary orbital retinoblastoma, enucleation is preferred if orbital component has resolved after chemoreduction with 3–6 cycles while exenteration is performed in case of residual orbital disease even after 6 cycles of neoadjuvant chemotherapy. In secondary orbital retinoblastoma which occurs as an orbital recurrence following uncomplicated enucleation, residual mass excision is performed after regression of orbital component, while exenteration is preferred if no resolution is observed in orbital component even after 6 cycles of chemotherapy. In cases of accidental orbital retinoblastoma in an eye with unsuspected retinoblastoma, enucleation with en bloc excision of overlying conjunctiva with 4 mm margin is performed at the intraocular surgical incision or biopsy site. Cases with clear corneal incision without breach in conjunctiva can be conservatively followed and may not need any further treatment after enucleation. Eyes with aseptic orbital cellulitis secondary to tumor necrosis, phthisical eyes with conjunctival fibrosis, and eyes with staphyloma are prone to inadvertent intraoperative perforation. If an extrascleral extension is macroscopically visualized during enucleation, meticulous excision of the nodule along with overlying tenon's capsule should be done. If optic nerve extension is suspected by thickening and inelasticity and short nerve stump (<10 mm) is obtained, meticulous orbital exploration should be conducted to further excise an extra length of optic nerve [96]. Post-enucleation full-thickness scleral infiltration, extrascleral extension, or optic nerve involvement up to the cut end on histopathology are classified as microscopic orbital retinoblastoma and similar multimodal orbital protocol is followed [9, 105, 106]. Biointegrated implants are generally avoided in orbital disease as the subsequent radiotherapy may compromise implant vascularization and increase the risk for implant exposure [98].

A study on stage III retinoblastoma (International Retinoblastoma Staging System) [7] showed that hematological toxicities were more common in children treated with five drugs' therapy carboplatin and etoposide, alternating with cyclophosphamide, idarubicin, and vincristine. They concluded that VEC protocol showed more effective tumor control and a better safety profile for nonmetastatic orbital retinoblastoma [107]. With multimodal treatment, survival of 50–70% is reported in patients with extraocular retinoblastoma [79].

Metastatic Retinoblastoma

Metastatic disease is common in developing countries with frequency ranging from 9 to 11% at presentation [108]. It usually occurs as a relapse following enucleation for intraocular retinoblastoma, especially in those who had high-risk pathologic features [109]. Most commonly, metastasis occurs in the central nervous system (CNS), bone (long bones–craniofacial bones), bone marrow, regional lymph nodes, orbit, and liver. Central nervous system (CNS) metastasis is the most common cause of relapse and death. Therefore it is mandatory to perform cerebrospinal fluid cytology, bone marrow evaluation, and whole-body imaging in all cases of metastatic retinoblastoma for disease staging.

Intensive chemotherapy including high-dose chemotherapy with autologous hematopoietic stem cell rescue has offered encouraging results with tumor control in 67% cases in stage 4a disease that does not involve the CNS [109]. Intensive treatment in the form of conventional induction chemotherapy with EBRT followed by escalated high-dose chemotherapy and autologous stem cell rescue has shown promising results in metastatic disease without CNS involvement but survival from CNS metastasis remains poor [110]. Additional craniospinal irradiation and intrathecal chemotherapy for CNS lesions have been recommended and found advantageous in stage 4b retinoblastoma (central nervous system metastatic disease) [111]. However, prognosis remains poor with event-free survival of 2/7 patients at 8-year follow-up [112]. Various regimens for induction therapy (vincristine, cyclophosphamide, cisplatin, and etoposide), high-dose chemotherapy (melphalan, cyclophosphamide, cisplatin, carboplatin, and thiotepa alone/with etoposide or topotecan), and intrathecal chemotherapy (methotrexate alone/with hydrocortisone and cytarabine) have been described in literature [109, 110].

Conclusion

In summary, retinoblastoma is curable if accurately diagnosed and appropriately managed in early stages. Introduction of newer treatment modalities and techniques has presented encouraging results in the tumor control. Continuous evolution and expansion of these modalities and their indications are indispensable in the conservative management of this malignancy for better treatment outcomes.

References

1. Shields JA, Shields CL. Intraocular tumors: a text and atlas. Philadelphia: WB Saunders; 1992.
2. Epstein JA, Shields CL, Shields JA. Trends in the management of retinoblastoma: evaluation of 1,196 consecutive eyes during 1974 to 2001. J Pediatr Ophthalmol Strabismus. 2003;40(4):196–203.
3. Shields CL, Shields JA. Retinoblastoma management: advances in enucleation, intravenous chemoreduction, and intra-arterial chemotherapy. Curr Opin Ophthalmol. 2010;21(3):203–12.
4. Linn MA. Intraocular retinoblastoma: the case for a new group classification. Ophthalmol Clin N Am. 2005;18(1):41–53. viii.
5. Shields CL, Mashayekhi A, Au AK, Czyz C, Leahey A, Meadows AT, et al. The international classification of retinoblastoma predicts chemoreduction success. Ophthalmology. 2006;113(12):2276–80.
6. Kaliki S, Shields CL, Rojanaporn D, Al-Dahmash S, McLaughlin JP, Shields JA, et al. High-risk retinoblastoma based on international classification of retinoblastoma: analysis of 519 enucleated eyes. Ophthalmology. 2013;120(5):997–1003.
7. Chantada G, Doz F, Antoneli CBG, Grundy R, Clare Stannard FF, Dunkel IJ, et al. A proposal for an international retinoblastoma staging system. Pediatr Blood Cancer. 2006;47(6):801–5.
8. Bakhshi S, Meel R, Kashyap S, Sharma S. Bone marrow aspirations and lumbar punctures in retinoblastoma at diagnosis: correlation with IRSS staging. J Pediatr Hematol Oncol. 2011;33(5):e182–5.
9. Honavar SG, Singh AD. Management of advanced retinoblastoma. Ophthalmol Clin. 2005;18(1):65–73.
10. Chawla B, Jain A, Azad R. Conservative treatment modalities in retinoblastoma. Indian J Ophthalmol. 2013;61(9):479–85.
11. Shields CL, Shields JA, Needle M, de Potter P, Kheterpal S, Hamada A, et al. Combined chemoreduction and adjuvant treatment for intraocular retinoblastoma. Ophthalmology. 1997;104(12):2101–11.
12. Shields CL, Fulco EM, Arias JD, Alarcon C, Pellegrini M, Rishi P, et al. Retinoblastoma frontiers with intravenous, intra-arterial, periocular, and intravitreal chemotherapy [Internet]. Eye. 2012. https://www.nature.com/articles/eye2012175. Accessed 15 Nov 2017.
13. Shields CL, Honavar SG, Meadows AT, Shields JA, Demirci H, Singh A, et al. Chemoreduction plus focal therapy for retinoblastoma: factors predictive of need for treatment with external beam radiotherapy or enucleation. Am J Ophthalmol. 2002;133(5):657–64.
14. Shields CL, De Potter P, Himelstein BP, Shields JA, Meadows AT, Maris JM. Chemoreduction in the initial management of intraocular retinoblastoma. Arch Ophthalmol. 1996;114(11):1330–8.
15. Wilson MW, Rodriguez-Galindo C, Haik BG, Moshfeghi DM, Merchant TE, Pratt CB. Multiagent chemotherapy as neoadjuvant treatment for multifocal intraocular retinoblastoma. Ophthalmology. 2001;108(11):2106–14. discussion 2114-2115.
16. Shields CL, Honavar SG, Shields JA, Demirci H, Meadows AT, Naduvilath TJ. Factors predictive of recurrence of retinal tumors, vitreous seeds, and subretinal seeds following chemoreduction for retinoblastoma. Arch Ophthalmol. 2002;120(4):460–4.
17. Shields CL, Mashayekhi A, Cater J, Shelil A, Meadows AT, Shields JA. Chemoreduction for retinoblastoma. Analysis of tumor control and risks for recurrence in 457 tumors. Am J Ophthalmol. 2004;138(3):329–37.
18. Dunkel IJ, Jubran RF, Gururangan S, Chantada GL, Finlay JL, Goldman S, et al. Trilateral retinoblastoma: potentially curable with intensive chemotherapy. Pediatr Blood Cancer. 2010;54(3):384–7.
19. Shields CL, Ramasubramanian A, Thangappan A, Hartzell K, Leahey A, Meadows AT, et al. Chemoreduction for group E retinoblastoma: comparison of chemoreduction alone versus chemoreduction plus low-dose external radiotherapy in 76 eyes. Ophthalmology. 2009;116(3):544–551.e1.

20. Kingston JE, Hungerford JL, Madreperla SA, Plowman PN. Results of combined chemotherapy and radiotherapy for advanced intraocular retinoblastoma. Arch Ophthalmol. 1996;114(11):1339–43.
21. Jenkinson H. Retinoblastoma: diagnosis and management—the UK perspective. Arch Dis Child. 2015;100(11):1070–5.
22. Abramson DH, Dunkel IJ, Brodie SE, Kim JW, Gobin YP. A phase I/II study of direct intra-arterial (ophthalmic artery) chemotherapy with melphalan for intraocular retinoblastoma: initial results. Ophthalmology. 2008;115(8):1398–404.
23. Kaneko A, Suzuki S. Eye-preservation treatment of retinoblastoma with vitreous seeding. Jpn J Clin Oncol. 2003;33(12):601–7.
24. Suzuki S, Kaneko A. Management of intraocular retinoblastoma and ocular prognosis. Int J Clin Oncol. 2004;9(1):1–6.
25. Shields CL, Jorge R, Say EAT, Magrath G, Alset A, Caywood E, et al. Unilateral retinoblastoma managed with intravenous chemotherapy versus intra-arterial chemotherapy. Outcomes based on the international classification of retinoblastoma. Asia Pac J Ophthalmol (Phila). 2016;5(2):97.
26. Shields CL, Manjandavida FP, Lally SE, Pieretti G, Arepalli SA, Caywood EH, et al. Intra-arterial chemotherapy for retinoblastoma in 70 eyes: outcomes based on the international classification of retinoblastoma. Ophthalmology. 2014;121(7):1453–60.
27. Tuncer S, Sencer S, Kebudi R, Tanyıldız B, Cebeci Z, Aydın K. Superselective intra-arterial chemotherapy in the primary management of advanced intra-ocular retinoblastoma: first 4-year experience from a single institution in Turkey. Acta Ophthalmol. 2016;94(7):e644–51.
28. Shields CL, Alset AE, Say EAT, Caywood E, Jabbour P, Shields JA. Retinoblastoma control with primary intra-arterial chemotherapy: outcomes before and during the intravitreal chemotherapy era. J Pediatr Ophthalmol Strabismus. 2016;53(5):275–84.
29. Say EAT, Iyer PG, Hasanreisoglu M, Lally SE, Jabbour P, Shields JA, et al. Secondary and tertiary intra-arterial chemotherapy for massive persistent or recurrent subretinal retinoblastoma seeds following previous chemotherapy exposure: long-term tumor control and globe salvage in 30 eyes. J AAPOS. 2016;20(4):337–42.
30. Muen WJ, Kingston JE, Robertson F, Brew S, Sagoo MS, Reddy MA. Efficacy and complications of super-selective intra-ophthalmic artery melphalan for the treatment of refractory retinoblastoma. Ophthalmology. 2012;119(3):611–6.
31. Gobin YP, Dunkel IJ, Marr BP, Brodie SE, Abramson DH. Intra-arterial chemotherapy for the management of retinoblastoma: four-year experience. Arch Ophthalmol. 2011;129(6):732–7.
32. Shields CL, Kaliki S, Al-Dahmash S, Rojanaporn D, Leahey A, Griffin G, et al. Management of advanced retinoblastoma with intravenous chemotherapy then intra-arterial chemotherapy as alternative to enucleation. Retina. 2013;33(10):2103.
33. Abramson DH, Marr BP, Dunkel IJ, Brodie S, Zabor EC, Driscoll SJ, et al. Intra-arterial chemotherapy for retinoblastoma in eyes with vitreous and/or subretinal seeding: 2-year results. Br J Ophthalmol. 2012;96(4):499–502.
34. Abramson DH, Marr BP, Francis JH, Dunkel IJ, Fabius AWM, Brodie SE, et al. Simultaneous bilateral ophthalmic artery chemosurgery for bilateral retinoblastoma (tandem therapy). PLoS One. 2016;11(6):e0156806.
35. Shields CL, Say EA, Pointdujour-Lim R, Cao C, Jabbour PM, Shields JA. Rescue intra-arterial chemotherapy following retinoblastoma recurrence after initial intra-arterial chemotherapy. J Fr Ophtalmol. 2015;38(6):542–9.
36. Leal-Leal CA, Asencio-López L, Higuera-Calleja J, Bernal-Moreno M, Bosch-Canto V, Chávez-Pacheco J, et al. Globe salvage with intra-arterial topotecan-melphalan chemotherapy in children with a single eye. Rev Invest Clin. 2016;68(3):137–42.
37. Chen M, Zhao J, Xia J, Liu Z, Jiang H, Shen G, et al. Intra-arterial chemotherapy as primary therapy for retinoblastoma in infants less than 3 months of age: a series of 10 case-studies. PLoS One. 2016;11(8):e0160873.

38. Magan T, Khoo CTL, Jabbour PM, Fuller DG, Shields CL. Intra-arterial chemotherapy for adult onset retinoblastoma in a 32-year-old man. J Pediatr Ophthalmol Strabismus. 2016;30(53):e43–6.
39. Rishi P, Sharma T, Koundanya V, Bansal N, Saravanan M, Ravikumar R, et al. Intra-arterial chemotherapy for retinoblastoma: first Indian report. Indian J Ophthalmol. 2015;63(4):331–4.
40. Shields CL, Ramasubramanian A, Rosenwasser R, Shields JA. Superselective catheterization of the ophthalmic artery for intra-arterial chemotherapy for retinoblastoma. Retina. 2009;29(8):1207–9.
41. Michaels ST, Abruzzo TA, Augsburger JJ, Corrêa ZM, Lane A, Geller JI. Selective ophthalmic artery infusion chemotherapy for advanced intraocular retinoblastoma: CCHMC early experience. J Pediatr Hematol Oncol. 2016;38(1):65–9.
42. Yannuzzi NA, Francis JH, Marr BP, Belinsky I, Dunkel IJ, Gobin YP, et al. Enucleation vs. ophthalmic artery chemosurgery for advanced intraocular retinoblastoma: a retrospective analysis. JAMA Ophthalmol. 2015;133(9):1062–6.
43. Simultaneous bilateral ophthalmic artery chemosurgery for bilateral retinoblastoma (tandem therapy). https://www.ncbi.nlm.nih.gov/pubmed/27258771. Accessed 8 Nov 2017.
44. Bertelli E, Leonini S, Galimberti D, Moretti S, Tinturini R, Hadjistilianou T, et al. Hemodynamic and anatomic variations require an adaptable approach during intra-arterial chemotherapy for intraocular retinoblastoma: alternative routes, strategies, and follow-up. Am J Neuroradiol. 2016;37(7):1289–95.
45. Chawla B, Singh R. Recent advances and challenges in the management of retinoblastoma. Indian J Ophthalmol. 2017;65(2):133.
46. Inomata M, Kaneko A. Chemosensitivity profiles of primary and cultured human retinoblastoma cells in a human tumor clonogenic assay. Jpn J Cancer Res. 1987;78(8):858–68.
47. Munier FL, Gaillard M-C, Balmer A, Soliman S, Podilsky G, Moulin AP, et al. Intravitreal chemotherapy for vitreous disease in retinoblastoma revisited: from prohibition to conditional indications. Br J Ophthalmol. 2012;96(8):1078–83.
48. Munier FL, Soliman S, Moulin AP, Gaillard M-C, Balmer A, Beck-Popovic M. Profiling safety of intravitreal injections for retinoblastoma using an anti-reflux procedure and sterilisation of the needle track. Br J Ophthalmol. 2012;96(8):1084–7.
49. Munier FL. Classification and management of seeds in retinoblastoma. Ellsworth Lecture Ghent August 24th 2013. Ophthalmic Genet. 2014;35(4):193–207.
50. Ghassemi F, Shields CL. Intravitreal melphalan for refractory or recurrent vitreous seeding from retinoblastoma. Arch Ophthalmol. 2012;130(10):1268–71.
51. Francis JH, Abramson DH, Gaillard M-C, Marr BP, Beck-Popovic M, Munier FL. The classification of vitreous seeds in retinoblastoma and response to intravitreal melphalan. Ophthalmology. 2015;122(6):1173–9.
52. Shields CL, Manjandavida FP, Arepalli S, Kaliki S, Lally SE, Shields JA. Intravitreal melphalan for persistent or recurrent retinoblastoma vitreous seeds: preliminary results. JAMA Ophthalmol. 2014;132(3):319–25.
53. Kaneko A. Treatment of vitreous seed of retinoblastoma recurrent after chemoreduction using vitreous injection of melphalan. World Congress of Ophthalmology. 2006.
54. Brodie SE, Munier FL, Francis JH, Marr B, Gobin YP, Abramson DH. Persistence of retinal function after intravitreal melphalan injection for retinoblastoma. Doc Ophthalmol. 2013;126(1):79–84.
55. Francis JH, Schaiquevich P, Buitrago E, Del Sole MJ, Zapata G, Croxatto JO, et al. Local and systemic toxicity of intravitreal melphalan for vitreous seeding in retinoblastoma: a preclinical and clinical study. Ophthalmology. 2014;121(9):1810–7.
56. Smith SJ, Smith BD, Mohney BG. Ocular side effects following intravitreal injection therapy for retinoblastoma: a systematic review. Br J Ophthalmol. 2014;98(3):292–7.
57. Ghassemi F, Shields CL, Ghadimi H, Khodabandeh A, Roohipoor R. Combined intravitreal melphalan and topotecan for refractory or recurrent vitreous seeding from retinoblastoma. JAMA Ophthalmol. 2014;132(8):936–41.
58. Abramson DH, Schefler AC. Update on retinoblastoma. Retina. 2004;24(6):828–48.

59. Mulvihill A, Budning A, Jay V, Vandenhoven C, Heon E, Gallie BL, et al. Ocular motility changes after subtenon carboplatin chemotherapy for retinoblastoma. Arch Ophthalmol. 2003;121(8):1120–4.
60. Abramson DH, Frank CM, Dunkel IJ. A phase I/II study of subconjunctival carboplatin for intraocular retinoblastoma. Ophthalmology. 1999;106(10):1947–50.
61. Shields CL, Shields JA. Diagnosis and management of retinoblastoma. Cancer Control. 2004;11(5):317–27.
62. Manjandavida FP, Honavar SG, Reddy VAP, Khanna R. Management and outcome of retinoblastoma with vitreous seeds. Ophthalmology. 2014;121(2):517–24.
63. Kang SJ, Durairaj C, Kompella UB, O'Brien JM, Liu K, Grossniklaus HE. Subconjunctival nanoparticle carboplatin in the treatment of transgenic murine retinoblastoma. Invest Ophthalmol Vis Sci. 2008;49(13):2017.
64. Kalita D, Shome D, Jain VG, Chadha K, Bellare JR. In vivo intraocular distribution and safety of periocular nanoparticle carboplatin for treatment of advanced retinoblastoma in humans. Am J Ophthalmol. 2014;157(5):1109–15.
65. Shah PK, Kalpana N, Narendran V, Ramakrishnan M. Severe aseptic orbital cellulitis with subtenon carboplatin for intraocular retinoblastoma. Indian J Ophthalmol. 2011;59(1):49–51.
66. Schmack I, Hubbard GB, Kang SJ, Aaberg TM, Grossniklaus HE. Ischemic necrosis and atrophy of the optic nerve after periocular carboplatin injection for intraocular retinoblastoma. Am J Ophthalmol. 2006;142(2):310–5.
67. Martin NE, Kim JW, Abramson DH. Fibrin sealant for retinoblastoma: where are we? J Ocul Pharmacol Ther. 2008;24(5):433–8.
68. Chawla B, Jain A, Seth R, Azad R, Mohan VK, Pushker N, et al. Clinical outcome and regression patterns of retinoblastoma treated with systemic chemoreduction and focal therapy: a prospective study. Indian J Ophthalmol. 2016;64(7):524.
69. Shields JA, Parsons H, Shields CL, Giblin ME. The role of cryotherapy in the management of retinoblastoma. Am J Ophthalmol. 1989;108(3):260–4.
70. Shields CL, Santos MCM, Diniz W, Gündüz K, Mercado G, Cater JR, et al. Thermotherapy for retinoblastoma. Arch Ophthalmol. 1999;117(7):885–93.
71. Shields CL, Shields JA, Kiratli H, De PP. Treatment of retinoblastoma with indirect ophthalmoscope laser photocoagulation. J Pediatr Ophthalmol Strabismus. 1995;32(5):317–22.
72. Shields CL, Mashayekhi A, Cater J, Shelil A, Ness S, Meadows AT, et al. Macular retinoblastoma managed with chemoreduction: analysis of tumor control with or without adjuvant thermotherapy in 68 tumors. Arch Ophthalmol. 2005;123(6):765–73.
73. Gombos DS, Kelly A, Coen PG, Kingston JE, Hungerford JL. Retinoblastoma treated with primary chemotherapy alone: the significance of tumour size, location, and age. Br J Ophthalmol. 2002;86(1):80–3.
74. Schefler AC, Cicciarelli N, Feuer W, Toledano S, Murray TG. Macular retinoblastoma: evaluation of tumor control, local complications, and visual outcomes for eyes treated with chemotherapy and repetitive foveal laser ablation. Ophthalmology. 2007;114(1):162–9.
75. Shields CL, Mashayekhi A, Sun H, Uysal Y, Friere J, Komarnicky L, et al. Iodine 125 plaque radiotherapy as salvage treatment for retinoblastoma recurrence after chemoreduction in 84 tumors. Ophthalmology. 2006;113(11):2087–92.
76. Schueler AO, Flühs D, Anastassiou G, Jurklies C, Sauerwein W, Bornfeld N. Beta-ray brachytherapy of retinoblastoma: feasibility of a new small-sized ruthenium-106 plaque. Ophthalmic Res. 2006;38(1):8–12.
77. Abouzeid H, Moeckli R, Gaillard M-C, Beck-Popovic M, Pica A, Zografos L, et al. 106Ruthenium brachytherapy for retinoblastoma. Int J Radiat Oncol Biol Phys. 2008;71(3):821–8.
78. Merchant TE, Gould CJ, Wilson MW, Hilton NE, Rodriguez-Galindo C, Haik BG. Episcleral plaque brachytherapy for retinoblastoma. Pediatr Blood Cancer. 2004;43(2):134–9.
79. Shields CL, Shields JA, De Potter P, Minelli S, Hernandez C, Brady LW, et al. Plaque radiotherapy in the management of retinoblastoma: use as a primary and secondary treatment. Ophthalmology. 1993;100(2):216–24.

80. Shields CL, Shields JA, Cater J, Othmane I, Singh AD, Micaily B. Plaque radiotherapy for retinoblastoma: long-term tumor control and treatment complications in 208 tumors. Ophthalmology. 2001;108(11):2116–21.
81. American Brachytherapy Society—Ophthalmic Oncology Task Force. Electronic address: paulfinger@eyecancer.com, ABS—OOTF Committee. The American Brachytherapy Society consensus guidelines for plaque brachytherapy of uveal melanoma and retinoblastoma. Brachytherapy. 2014;13(1):1–14.
82. Eldebawy E, Parker W, Abdel Rahman W, Freeman CR. Dosimetric study of current treatment options for radiotherapy in retinoblastoma. Int J Radiat Oncol Biol Phys. 2012;82(3):e501–5.
83. Eldebawy E, Patrocinio H, Evans M, Hashem R, Nelson S, Sidi R, et al. Stereotactic radiotherapy as an alternative to plaque brachytherapy in retinoblastoma. Pediatr Blood Cancer. 2010;55(6):1210–2.
84. Sethi RV, Shih HA, Yeap BY, Mouw KW, Petersen R, Kim DY, et al. Second nonocular tumors among survivors of retinoblastoma treated with contemporary photon and proton radiotherapy. Cancer. 2014;120(1):126–33.
85. Kaliki S, Srinivasan V, Gupta A, Mishra DK, Naik MN. Clinical features predictive of high-risk retinoblastoma in 403 Asian Indian patients: a case-control study. Ophthalmology. 2015;122(6):1165–72.
86. Mudhar S, Brundler MA, Luthert P. Standards and datasets for reporting cancers. Dataset for ocular retinoblastoma histopathology reports. Rep R Coll Pathol. 2010.
87. Messmer EP, Heinrich T, Höpping W, de Sutter E, Havers W, Sauerwein W. Risk factors for metastases in patients with retinoblastoma. Ophthalmology. 1991;98(2):136–41.
88. Shields CL, Shields JA, Baez KA, Cater J, De Potter PV. Choroidal invasion of retinoblastoma: metastatic potential and clinical risk factors. Br J Ophthalmol. 1993;77(9):544–8.
89. Shields CL, Shields JA, Baez K, Cater JR, De Potter P. Optic nerve invasion of retinoblastoma. Metastatic potential and clinical risk factors. Cancer. 1994;73(3):692–8.
90. Eagle RC Jr. High-risk features and tumor differentiation in retinoblastoma: a retrospective histopathologic study. Arch Pathol Lab Med. 2009;133(8):1203–9.
91. Uusitalo MS, Van Quill KR, Scott IU, Matthay KK, Murray TG, O'brien JM. Evaluation of chemoprophylaxis in patients with unilateral retinoblastoma with high-risk features on histopathologic examination. Arch Ophthalmol. 2001;119(1):41–8.
92. Honavar SG, Singh AD, Shields CL, Meadows AT, Demirci H, Cater J, et al. Postenucleation adjuvant therapy in high-risk retinoblastoma. Arch Ophthalmol. 2002;120(7):923–31.
93. Chantada GL, Casco F, Fandiño AC, Galli S, Manzitti J, Scopinaro M, et al. Outcome of patients with retinoblastoma and postlaminar optic nerve invasion. Ophthalmology. 2007;114(11):2083–9.
94. Honavar SG. Orbital retinoblastoma. In: Clinical ophthalmic oncology [Internet]. Berlin: Springer; 2015. p. 185–94. https://link.springer.com/chapter/10.1007/978-3-662-43451-2_17. Accessed 18 Nov 2017.
95. Chawla B, Hasan F, Azad R, Seth R, Upadhyay AD, Pathy S, et al. Clinical presentation and survival of retinoblastoma in Indian children. Br J Ophthalmol. 2016;100(2):172–8.
96. Ali MJ, Honavar SG, Reddy VAP. Orbital retinoblastoma: present status and future challenges—a review. Saudi J Ophthalmol. 2011;25(2):159–67.
97. Badhu B, Sah SP, Thakur SK, Dulal S, Kumar S, Sood A, et al. Clinical presentation of retinoblastoma in Eastern Nepal. Clin Exp Ophthalmol. 2005;33(4):386–9.
98. Honavar SG, Manjandavida FP, Reddy VAP. Orbital retinoblastoma: an update. Indian J Ophthalmol. 2017;65(6):435–42.
99. Gündüz K, Müftüoglu O, Günalp I, Unal E, Taçyildiz N. Metastatic retinoblastoma clinical features, treatment, and prognosis. Ophthalmology. 2006;113(9):1558–66.
100. Moll AC, Hoekstra OS, Imhof SM, Comans EF, Schouten-van Meeteren AYN, van der Valk P, et al. Fluorine-18 fluorodeoxyglucose positron emission tomography (PET) to detect vital retinoblastoma in the eye: preliminary experience. Ophthalmic Genet. 2004;25(1):31–5.
101. Kiratli PO, Kiratli H, Ercan MT. Visualization of orbital retinoblastoma with technetium-99m (V) dimercaptosuccinic acid. Ann Nucl Med. 1998;12(3):157–9.

102. Antoneli CBG, Steinhorst F, de Cássia Braga Ribeiro K, PERS N, MMM C, Arias V, et al. Extraocular retinoblastoma: a 13-year experience. Cancer. 2003;98(6):1292–8.
103. Chantada G, Fandiño A, Casak S, Manzitti J, Raslawski E, Schvartzman E. Treatment of overt extraocular retinoblastoma. Med Pediatr Oncol. 2003;40(3):158–61.
104. Chantada GL, Guitter MR, Fandiño AC, Raslawski EC, de Davila MTG, Vaiani E, et al. Treatment results in patients with retinoblastoma and invasion to the cut end of the optic nerve. Pediatr Blood Cancer. 2009;52(2):218–22.
105. Finger PT, Harbour JW, Karcioglu ZA. Risk factors for metastasis in retinoblastoma. Surv Ophthalmol. 2002;47(1):1–16.
106. Singh AD, Shields CL, Shields JA. Prognostic factors in retinoblastoma. J Pediatr Ophthalmol Strabismus. 2000;37(3):134–41. quiz 168-169.
107. Chawla B, Hasan F, Seth R, Pathy S, Pattebahadur R, Sharma S, et al. Multimodal therapy for stage III retinoblastoma (international retinoblastoma staging system): a prospective comparative study. Ophthalmology. 2016;123(9):1933–9.
108. Ali MJ, Honavar SG, Reddy VA. Distant metastatic retinoblastoma without central nervous system involvement. Indian J Ophthalmol. 2013;61(7):357–9.
109. Dunkel IJ, Khakoo Y, Kernan NA, Gershon T, Gilheeney S, Lyden DC, et al. Intensive multimodality therapy for patients with stage 4a metastatic retinoblastoma. Pediatr Blood Cancer. 2010;55(1):55–9.
110. Matsubara H, Makimoto A, Higa T, Kawamoto H, Sakiyama S, Hosono A, et al. A multidisciplinary treatment strategy that includes high-dose chemotherapy for metastatic retinoblastoma without CNS involvement. Bone Marrow Transplant. 2005;35(8):763–6.
111. Malik M, Prabhakar R, Sharma DN, Rath GK. Retinoblastoma with cerebrospinal fluid metastasis treated with orbital and craniospinal irradiation using IMRT. Technol Cancer Res Treat. 2006;5(5):497–501.
112. Dunkel IJ, Chan HSL, Jubran R, Chantada GL, Goldman S, Chintagumpala M, et al. High-dose chemotherapy with autologous hematopoietic stem cell rescue for stage 4B retinoblastoma. Pediatr Blood Cancer. 2010;55(1):149–52.

Diagnosis and Management of Small Choroidal Melanoma

Amy C. Schefler and Ryan Sangwoo Kim

Introduction

Uveal melanoma is rare, but is the most common type of primary intraocular cancer in adults, and occurs in approximately six people per million annually in the United States [1]. Classically, most uveal melanomas are caused by sporadic mutations in melanocytes of the uvea and occur predominantly in non-Hispanic-Caucasian populations. Except for very rare cases of bilateral disease (mostly due to germline mutations), uveal melanoma is generally unilateral. Ninety percent of uveal melanomas arise in the choroid, while the remaining cases originate from the iris or ciliary body [2]. Despite its rarity, uveal melanoma can be highly malignant and metastasize in up to 50% of the cases via hematogenous route to the liver, lungs, and soft tissue (in the order of prevalence), with a mean post-metastatic survival of under a year [3–6]. Therefore, close monitoring of the disease progression once a clinical diagnosis is made as well as early medical intervention are critical for maximizing patient survival. Among available treatment modalities for choroidal melanoma, plaque brachytherapy, proton beam radiation, and enucleation are the accepted treatment options. Treatment is chosen based on various factors including tumor size and location, patient needs, and treatment costs. In this chapter, we discuss recent treatment advancements and current research in this disease.

A. C. Schefler (✉)
Retina Consultants of Houston, Blanton Eye Institute, Houston Methodist Hospital, Houston, TX, USA

Children's Memorial Hermann Hospital, University of Texas Health Sciences, San Antonio, TX, USA
e-mail: acsmd@houstonretina.com

R. S. Kim
Children's Memorial Hermann Hospital, University of Texas Health Sciences, San Antonio, TX, USA

© Springer Nature Singapore Pte Ltd. 2019
A. Ramasubramanian (ed.), *Ocular Oncology*, Current Practices in Ophthalmology, https://doi.org/10.1007/978-981-13-7538-5_2

Prognostic Markers Allowing for Patient-Specific Disease Management

Uveal melanoma is microscopically characterized by well-differentiated spindle-type cells or poorly differentiated epithelioid cells. Although uveal melanoma with epithelioid cell proliferation has been traditionally considered to be a more aggressive type, the majority of tumors contain mixed cell types. Therefore, it is difficult to determine specific tumor behaviors solely based on the histopathologic findings, as there are other factors that are also involved in the development of uveal melanoma. Ciliary body involvement has been understood to be correlated to worse prognosis and higher metastatic risk, largely due to rich vascularization in the ciliary body region that allows for rapid hematogenous dissemination of tumor cells to distal sites [7–9]. In contrast, iris tumors have lower metastatic potential than choroidal and ciliary body lesions and are often surgically resected [8]. Patient age is closely associated with prognosis, as multiple studies have demonstrated that older age at diagnosis corresponds to higher metastasis and disease-related death [10, 11].

Significant discoveries have been made since the early 2000s especially regarding the cytogenetic and molecular aspects of uveal melanoma that have allowed clinicians to categorize tumors based on metastatic potential. Molecular characterization of these tumors utilizing RNA-based tests such as genetic expression profiling (GEP) or DNA-based tests such as multiplex ligation-dependent probe amplification (MLPA) of uveal melanoma has become indispensable in the management of uveal melanoma. GEP has been demonstrated in randomized clinical trials to accurately classify tumors into either Class 1, which corresponds to a low metastatic risk, or Class 2 that has high metastatic risk [12]. Class 1 can be subdivided into 1A, whose metastatic risk remains steady over time, and 1B, which displays a gradually increasing metastatic risk. Overall reported 5-year metastatic risks for Class 1A, Class 1B, and Class 2 tumors are 2%, 21%, and 72%, respectively [13]. Most ocular oncologists now build patient-specific treatment regimens based on the molecular characteristics of each tumor.

Choroidal Nevus vs. Melanoma

It is important that clinicians accurately distinguish choroidal nevi from melanomas. Key clinical features, including tumor thickness greater than 2 mm, presence of fluid, orange pigmentation, hollowness on ultrasound, within 3 mm proximity to the optic disc, and absence of halo and drusen, have conventionally been used to make the distinction [14, 15]. Classically, if lesions possessed more than three of these risk factors, then they would be considered melanomas and managed accordingly (Figs. 1 and 2). However, a recent publication by Nguyen et al. reported that there may be a discrepancy between clinical risk factors of choroidal lesions and their GEP class, which is currently the most accurate marker for

Fig. 1 Fundus photograph of the left eye of a 71-year-old male patient demonstrating an elevated amelanotic lesion in the periphery with pigmentary changes. Tumor thickness was 2.44 mm at initial diagnosis, and the lesion was 2.2 mm away from the optic nerve, meeting the clinical definition of uveal melanoma. Upon subsequent GEP analysis, the patient's tumor was classified as Class 1A

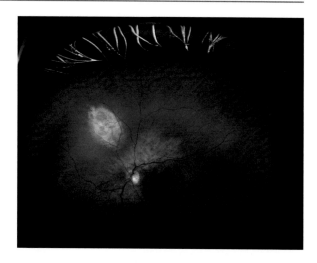

Fig. 2 B-scan ultrasound of the same eye of the same patient in Fig. 1, demonstrating a dome-shaped lesion in the posterior region. Note mild subretinal fluid over the apex of the lesion and mild-to-moderate vascularity in the image

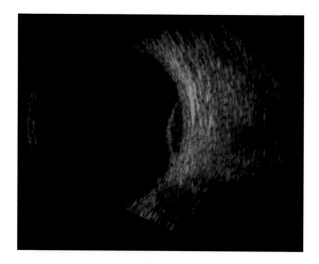

prognosis. Other similar studies from multiple institutions are currently in press. In this study, only American Joint Committee on Cancer (AJCC) tumor staging and LBD had statistically significant associations with higher GEP class [16]. This result suggests that a nevus lacking key risk factors could be molecularly classified as a GEP Class 2 tumor, or, conversely, a highly malignant-appearing lesion could be a nevus with little likelihood of becoming cancer. Large collaborative series of patients such as the Collaborative Ocular Oncology Group 2 (COOG2) will assess these classical risk factors in patients with large nevi/small melanomas in the coming years, helping clinicians to optimize their approach to the treatment of these lesions.

Importance of Fine-Needle Aspiration Biopsy

With the increasing importance of molecular analysis of uveal melanoma tumor cells for prognosis, numerous reports have been published on the techniques and safety of fine-needle aspiration biopsy (FNAB) of uveal melanoma tumor cells. FNAB is commonly used to harvest cells via a transscleral or transvitreal route, depending on the tumor geometry and location (Fig. 3). Most tumors located behind the equator are accessed transvitreally using standard retinal instrumentation, while anterior tumors allow for direct needle access through the underlying sclera. Multiple publications, including a histopathologic analysis of biopsy needle tracts that were created in vivo [17, 18], have demonstrated that extraocular spreading of tumor cells during the biopsy process is a truly rare event. Furthermore, numerous manuscripts have reported on the FNAB yield rates for subsequent cytopathologic and cytogenetic analyses, and many experienced centers surpass a yield rate of 80% [19–21].

For transscleral biopsy, transillumination is used to mark the border of the tumor on the sclera. Apical height of the tumor, which is obtained from B-scan ultrasound, is marked on the biopsy needle. The needle is then inserted, and cells are collected

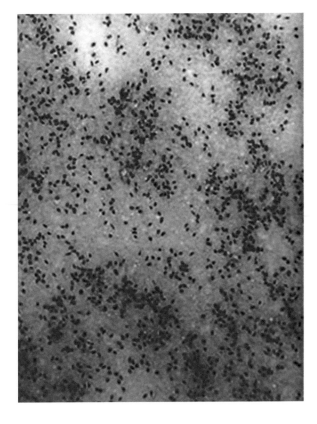

Fig. 3 A representative image of an adequacy slide that was prepared intraoperatively to assess the presence of tumor cells in the acquired fine-needle aspiration biopsy (FNAB) sample. Subsequent gene expression profile analysis categorizes tumors based on metastatic risk. Low-risk tumors are classified as Class 1, while high-risk tumors are classified as Class 2

using a biopsy aspiration gun. Once the biopsy procedure is complete, cryotherapy is performed at the needle insertion site to prevent any extraocular extension of tumor cells.

For transvitreal biopsy, indirect ophthalmoscopy or standard retinal instrumentation and chandelier light are used for direct visualization of the tumor. If retinal instrumentation is used, a trocar is placed on the opposite clock position from the tumor through which a long biopsy needle with a short bevel is placed to fully embed the needle within the tumor. Cells are aspirated by the biopsy gun. Cryotherapy of the needle insertion site is again performed. If it is a small lesion, a combination of a needle and a cutter can be used to increase the biopsy yield. Experienced centers are routinely able to get valuable molecular information from even small tumors with apical heights less than 3.0 mm [22].

Plaque Brachytherapy

Plaque brachytherapy was first introduced in the 1930s and, along with enucleation, has been used to treat intraocular malignancies. Plaque therapy, compared to enucleation, has a distinctive benefit of preserving the globe and possibly sparing patient vision. However, the first prospective randomized trial comparing these therapies did not occur until several decades later. The Collaborative Ocular Melanoma Study (COMS), which included a series of multicenter randomized clinical trials for small-, medium-, and large-sized melanomas, was initiated in the 1980s to analyze the critical clinical questions related to uveal melanoma at the time. The medium-sized tumor study was designed to compare the treatment efficacy and melanoma-specific mortality rates of patients who were randomly assigned to either enucleation or iodine-125 plaque radiotherapy as primary therapy for uveal melanoma. The study found that melanoma-specific mortality rates were statistically equivalent between the enucleation and brachytherapy groups [5]. Since the publication of this study, most patients with tumors amenable to plaque therapy have chosen this ocular- and in many cases vision-sparing treatment given the results of this trial. Nonetheless, visual loss after plaques can be significant. In a separate report on visual acuity published from the COMS data set, approximately half of the brachytherapy patients lost six or more lines of visual acuity from baseline at 3 years post-brachytherapy, while the percentage of patients having 20/200 or worse of visual acuity rose from 10% prior to therapy to 43% post-therapy [23]. Factors predicting vision loss including foveal involvement, large tumor apical height, tumor-related retinal detachment (RD), and a history of diabetes corresponded to worse clinical outcomes [23].

The results from the COMS trial led to a widespread adoption of plaque brachytherapy as the most commonly used primary treatment modality for uveal melanoma in the United States. Currently, three radioisotopes that are most commonly used for brachytherapy are ruthenium (^{106}Ru), iodine (^{125}I), and palladium (^{103}Pd). Iodine-125 is most frequently used in the United States, while ruthenium-106 is more commonly used in European countries. A detailed guideline for plaque therapy including standard dosage recommendation has been published by the American Brachytherapy Society [24, 25]. Currently, standard plaque therapy guidelines suggest prescribing a radiation dose of 85 Gy to the tumor's apical height or 5 mm from the inner scleral base (whichever is greater) for 5–12 days, with 7 days (168 h) being most conventional. A safety margin of 2 mm around the lesion is factored in when choosing the plaque design in order to ensure full coverage of the lesion, although 1 mm margin can be safely handled by some experienced centers. Compared to the COMS plaques, newer plaque designs including the Eye Physics plaque offer thinner and more customized profiles to better conform to each tumor's shape and size [26]. These features result in better shielding of surrounding healthy tissues from radiation exposure and a more focused and even distribution of the radiation dosage to the tumor.

Efficacy of plaque brachytherapy for the management of primary uveal melanoma has been repeatedly verified in the scientific literature, with local control rates often exceeding 95% [27–29]. A recent study reported that Class 1 tumors appear to respond better to plaque brachytherapy than their Class 2 counterparts and regress faster within the first 6 months after brachytherapy [30], which may provide useful prognostic information in patients who have not had gene expression profiling before therapy. Active investigations are currently being performed to delineate the relationship between GEP signature and patient response to brachytherapy.

The most feared complication of plaque brachytherapy is local recurrence of the tumor, as the possibility of systemic metastasis increases significantly after failure of local tumor control [31]. A recent publication of 3809 patients with uveal melanoma reported that patients with no local recurrence of the tumor had 5-year and 10-year metastasis-free Kaplan-Meier estimates of 87% and 82%, respectively [32]. In comparison, patients with local recurrence had 71% and 62% 5-year and 10-year metastasis-free survival rates, respectively, both of which were statistically significantly lower than those of the no-recurrence group. Therefore, achieving local control of the tumor is critical in helping to prevent metastasis. Recurrence can occur at central, distal, or marginal locations of the original tumor, and can be treated with salvage plaque therapy, transpupillary thermotherapy (TTT), or enucleation. Plaque as salvage therapy serves as a viable treatment option for locally recurrent tumors, and one study reported an overall control rate of 77% by Kaplan-Meier estimate when marginally and diffusely recurrent tumors were treated with subsequent salvage brachytherapy [27].

Whereas the rate of local recurrence in the COMS report was approximately 10% [33], several recent publications on the efficacy and safety of plaque brachytherapy report local recurrence rates below 5% [34, 35]. Several published approaches to surgery have aided in improving these results. First, increased use of intraoperative ultrasound to confirm the plaque position helps in ensuring that the plaque fully covers all tumor margins and that full targeted radiation dosage is delivered to the entirety of the tumor (Fig. 4) [35]. The rate of treatment failure is consistently below 2% in recent studies that utilized ultrasound confirmation of plaque position [28, 29, 35, 36]. Second, customization of the plaque design and seed configuration as well as rigorous treatment planning allow for precisely targeted dose of radiation. Tumors that were previously difficult to access, such as peripapillary

Fig. 4 Intraoperative B-scan ultrasound image immediately after the insertion of a plaque, demonstrating that the plaque has fully covered the tumor margins. Intraoperative ultrasound confirmation is now widely used to ensure precise plaque positioning

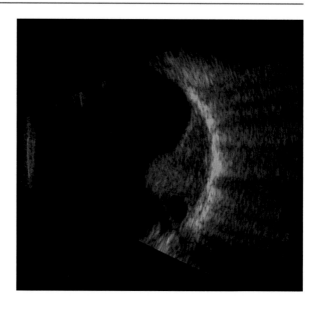

lesions, can now be managed with notched plaques that wrap around the optic nerve. Various Eye Physics and notched COMS plaque shapes are available to fit different tumor profiles.

Proton Beam Radiation

Proton beam radiation therapy is another viable treatment option for uveal melanoma. Although it is not as commonly used for primary therapy as plaque brachytherapy due to patient access, proton beam therapy has a published 4% local recurrence rate over more than 10 years [37, 38], which is comparable to that of plaque therapy. One key difference between proton beam radiation and plaque brachytherapy is that the affected eye is not fully stationary during the proton beam therapy, while the episcleral plaque is sutured to the sclera and remains in the same position for the duration of radiation. This can not only radiate the surrounding healthy tissue, but also lead to a possibility of some areas within the tumor not receiving the full calculated radiation dosage. Therefore, it is imperative to prescribe extra 2–3 mm of margin around the tumor in order for the protons to fully encompass the target region.

Complications After Radiation

Ocular complications including cataract, glaucoma, optic neuropathy, and radiation retinopathy can commonly arise after plaque brachytherapy and charged particle therapy (Fig. 5) [2, 39]. Additionally, certain superiorly located tumors treated by proton beam radiation can be accompanied by damage to the eyelid, which can

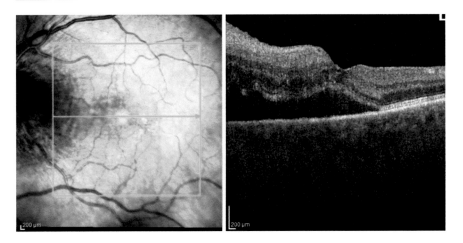

Fig. 5 Optical coherence tomography (OCT) image of the same eye in Fig. 1, 2 years post-plaque brachytherapy, demonstrating radiation-induced retinopathy. Note focal RPE elevations as well as retinal elevation that is consistent with subretinal fluid. Radiation retinopathy can commonly occur after either proton beam radiation or plaque therapy and can be managed with intravitreal anti-VEGF injections

manifest as keratinization of the palpebral conjunctiva and keratitis [2]. Irradiation can also cause radiation retinopathy which can subsequently lead to cystoid macular edema, exudation, ischemia, vitreous hemorrhage, and neovascular glaucoma [2]. Laser photocoagulation, anti-VEGF (vascular endothelial growth factor) injections, or intraocular steroids can be used to treat these ocular complications. Multiple retrospective studies have been published demonstrating the efficacy of anti-VEGF therapy for radiation retinopathy [40, 41]. One prospective trial has also been published demonstrating an improvement in vision compared to historical controls in patients treated with ranibizumab every 2 months after proton beam therapy [42]. Our center is currently conducting multiple prospective clinical trials examining the efficacy of anti-VEGF injections for radiation retinopathy for patients treated with iodine-125 plaques.

Other Therapy Options

Despite excellent clinical outcomes of enucleation, plaque brachytherapy, and proton bream radiation as primary treatment modalities, approximately half of uveal melanoma patients eventually develop metastasis [6], most frequently in the liver. Median survival for patients with widespread metastatic disease is less than a year. Many clinical trials for adjuvant or metastatic uveal melanoma therapies have either been conducted or are currently being performed, but there is not yet an FDA-approved treatment option that shows promising clinical results in an adjuvant or metastatic setting [43]. As for adjuvant therapy for uveal melanoma, several chemotherapeutic and immunomodulating agents including dacarbazine, interferon, and bacille Calmette-Guerin (BCG) have been previously tested in randomized clinical trials, only to yield no significant treatment benefits [44, 45]. Scientists are investigating standard alkylating or platinum compounds, monoclonal antibodies, vaccines, HDAC inhibitors, and MAPK inhibitors (as *GNAQ* and *GNA11* mutations lead to upregulation of the MAPK pathway) as therapeutic possibilities [44]. Currently, adjuvant clinical trials using valproic acid (NCT02068586), dacarbazine and interferon alfa-2b (NCT01100528), and dendritic cell vaccination (NCT01983748) are active.

For metastatic therapy, researchers focus on targeting the immune escape mechanism exhibited by uveal melanoma cells. Programmed cell death ligand-1 (PD-L1) can induce apoptosis in T cells that express PD-1 receptors. Thus, PD-L1 and PD-1 interaction allows tumor cells to avoid the immunologic attack by T cells [46]. Atezolizumab, pembrolizumab, and nivolumab are human monoclonal antibodies that block either PD-L1 or PD-1 receptor and subsequently inhibit the apoptosis of tumor-specific T cells. Cytotoxic T-lymphocyte-associated antigen 4 (CTLA-4) is also involved in immune checkpoint, and ipilimumab is another human monoclonal antibody specifically directed against CTLA-4. These immune checkpoint inhibitors have shown moderate efficacy for metastatic and/or cutaneous melanomas, but none have shown definitive clinical benefits for metastatic uveal melanoma [47, 48]. Many of the currently active studies are using combinations of these antibodies for potential therapeutic benefits.

Field et al. reported that some Class 1 tumors that eventually metastasized demonstrated mRNA overexpression of preferentially expressed antigen in melanoma (*PRAME*), which is a type of cancer-testis antigen that is normally not expressed in healthy adults [49]. This key finding of *PRAME* as an independent marker for metastasis is the first explanation of metastatic susceptibility in a small subset of Class 1 tumors. Some Class 2 tumors also exhibit *PRAME* activity, and it is currently theorized that *PRAME* expression in Class 2 tumors may accelerate the progression to metastasis. Gezgin et al. recently published that *PRAME* could be a potential target for immunotherapy, as *PRAME*-specific T cells reacted to melanomas with *PRAME* expression. Some metastatic melanoma samples expressed *PRAME* alone, HLA class 1 alone, or a combination of both. As healthy adult tissues normally do not express *PRAME*, if cytotoxic T cells can be specifically targeted from *PRAME*-expressed metastatic tumor cells, a new targeted immunotherapy might become possible [50].

Recently, a light-activated drug named AU-011 has been developed and is currently being tested in a Phase 1b/2 clinical trial. AU-011 conjugates HPV-like particles with a phthalocyanine photosensitizer so that the drug will uniquely bind the heparan sulfate proteoglycans that are abundantly expressed on tumor cells. When AU-011 receives near-infrared light, the drug's cytotoxic effect is activated and selectively kills uveal melanoma tumor cells [51]. AU-011 has received an orphan drug designation and is being actively investigated for a possible use as targeted therapy for uveal melanoma. The biggest advantage of this highly selective therapy is that it minimizes damages to surrounding healthy tissues to which the nanoparticles would not bind, allowing for maximal preservation of patient vision.

In summary, although local therapy for uveal melanoma has been refined and improved, the current status of adjuvant and metastatic therapies is yet empirical without promising outcomes. As the genetic and molecular details of uveal melanoma are better understood over time, researchers will focus on developing new treatments that can potentially prevent progression to metastasis and maximize patient survival. Further clinical trials may offer deeper insights into immunologic mechanisms of uveal melanoma and potential treatment solutions.

Current Pearls and Pitfalls

- Despite therapeutic efforts, approximately 50% of uveal melanomas progress to metastatic disease; once the disease metastasizes, patient survival greatly decreases. There are currently no treatments available to successfully manage metastatic uveal melanoma.
- The COMS clinical trial since the 1980s shifted the paradigm of management of uveal melanoma. COMS reports demonstrated that patients treated with plaque brachytherapy had a comparable mortality rate to those who underwent enucleation as primary treatment. This outcome led to a widespread adoption of plaque brachytherapy as the most commonly prescribed treatment for uveal melanoma.
- Plaque brachytherapy has demonstrated superior management of primary uveal melanomas. Local recurrence rate in recent publication has been consistently low at 0–3%, especially with the use of intraoperative ultrasound for the confirmation of plaque position.
- Since the introduction of GEP testing, molecular analysis of uveal melanoma has allowed for classification of patients based on metastatic risk (low-risk Class 1 vs. high-risk Class 2). Class 1 has been subdivided into 1A (metastatic risk remains low over time) and 1B (metastatic risk increases over time). Molecular classification of uveal melanoma allows clinicians to design a tumor- and patient-specific treatment regimen.
- As the importance of genomic analysis has increased, techniques to safely and precisely collect tumor samples via FNAB have become crucial. There are multiple reports that validate the safety of the FNAB procedure as well as offer techniques to increase biopsy yield.
- Studies are being conducted to elucidate a clear association between GEP signature and treatment outcomes. Notably, a recent collaborative study reported that Class 1 tumors regress faster than Class 2 tumors after plaque therapy.
- *PRAME* expression has recently been discovered to play a significant role in causing metastasis in Class 1 tumors as well as accelerating metastatic process in Class 2 tumors.
- Multiple studies are investigating uveal melanoma-targeted immunotherapies using CTLA-4 and PD-1/PD-L1 antibodies. Although no definitive benefits have been discovered yet, future studies may provide insights into potential ways to manage metastatic uveal melanoma.

References

1. Hu DN, Yu GP, McCormick SA, Schneider S, Finger PT. Population-based incidence of uveal melanoma in various races and ethnic groups. Am J Ophthalmol. 2005;140(4):612–7. https://doi.org/10.1016/j.ajo.2005.05.034.
2. Dogrusoz M, Jager MJ, Damato B. Uveal melanoma treatment and prognostication. Asia Pac J Ophthalmol. 2017;6(2):186–96. https://doi.org/10.22608/APO.201734.
3. Collaborative Ocular Melanoma Study Group. Assessment of metastatic disease status at death in 435 patients with large choroidal melanoma in the Collaborative Ocular Melanoma Study (COMS): COMS report no. 15. Arch Ophthalmol. 2001;119(5):670–6.
4. Diener-West M, Reynolds SM, Agugliaro DJ, Caldwell R, Cumming K, Earle JD, Hawkins BS, Hayman JA, Jaiyesimi I, Jampol LM, Kirkwood JM, Koh WJ, Robertson DM, Shaw JM, Straatsma BR, Thoma J, Collaborative Ocular Melanoma Study Group. Development of metastatic disease after enrollment in the COMS trials for treatment of choroidal melanoma: Collaborative Ocular Melanoma Study Group report no. 26. Arch Ophthalmol. 2005;123(12):1639–43. https://doi.org/10.1001/archopht.123.12.1639.
5. Diener-West M, Earle JD, Fine SL, Hawkins BS, Moy CS, Reynolds SM, Schachat AP, Straatsma BR, Collaborative Ocular Melanoma Study Group. The COMS randomized trial of iodine 125 brachytherapy for choroidal melanoma, III: initial mortality findings. COMS report no. 18. Arch Ophthalmol. 2001;119(7):969–82.
6. Kujala E, Makitie T, Kivela T. Very long-term prognosis of patients with malignant uveal melanoma. Invest Ophthalmol Vis Sci. 2003;44(11):4651–9.
7. Chew AL, Spilsbury K, Isaacs TW. Survival from uveal melanoma in Western Australia 1981-2005. Clin Exp Ophthalmol. 2015;43(5):422–8. https://doi.org/10.1111/ceo.12490.
8. Shields CL, Furuta M, Thangappan A, Nagori S, Mashayekhi A, Lally DR, Kelly CC, Rudich DS, Nagori AV, Wakade OA, Mehta S, Forte L, Long A, Dellacava EF, Kaplan B, Shields JA. Metastasis of uveal melanoma millimeter-by-millimeter in 8033 consecutive eyes. Arch Ophthalmol. 2009;127(8):989–98. https://doi.org/10.1001/archophthalmol.2009.208.
9. Costache M, Patrascu OM, Adrian D, Costache D, Sajin M, Ungureanu E, Simionescu O. Ciliary body melanoma—a particularly rare type of ocular tumor. Case report and general considerations. Maedica (Buchar). 2013;8(4):360–4.
10. Shields CL, Kaliki S, Furuta M, Mashayekhi A, Shields JA. Clinical spectrum and prognosis of uveal melanoma based on age at presentation in 8,033 cases. Retina. 2012;32(7):1363–72. https://doi.org/10.1097/IAE.0b013e31824d09a8.
11. Kaliki S, Shields CL, Mashayekhi A, Ganesh A, Furuta M, Shields JA. Influence of age on prognosis of young patients with uveal melanoma: a matched retrospective cohort study. Eur J Ophthalmol. 2013;23(2):208–16. https://doi.org/10.5301/ejo.5000200.
12. Onken MD, Worley LA, Ehlers JP, Harbour JW. Gene expression profiling in uveal melanoma reveals two molecular classes and predicts metastatic death. Cancer Res. 2004;64(20):7205–9. https://doi.org/10.1158/0008-5472.CAN-04-1750.
13. Field MG, Harbour JW. Recent developments in prognostic and predictive testing in uveal melanoma. Curr Opin Ophthalmol. 2014;25(3):234–9. https://doi.org/10.1097/ICU.0000000000000051.
14. Shields CL, Kels JG, Shields JA. Melanoma of the eye: revealing hidden secrets, one at a time. Clin Dermatol. 2015;33(2):183–96. https://doi.org/10.1016/j.clindermatol.2014.10.010.
15. The Collaborative Ocular Melanoma Study Group. Factors predictive of growth and treatment of small choroidal melanoma: COMS report no. 5. Arch Ophthalmol. 1997;115(12):1537–44.
16. Nguyen BT, Kim RS, Bretana ME, Kegley E, Schefler AC. Association between traditional clinical high-risk features and gene expression profile classification in uveal melanoma. Graefes Arch Clin Exp Ophthalmol. 2018;256(2):421–7. https://doi.org/10.1007/s00417-017-3856-x.
17. Kim RS, Chevez-Barrios P, Bretana ME, Wong TP, Teh BS, Schefler AC. Histopathologic analysis of transvitreal fine needle aspiration biopsy needle tracts for uveal melanoma. Am J Ophthalmol. 2017;174:9–16. https://doi.org/10.1016/j.ajo.2016.10.019.

18. Schefler AC, Gologorsky D, Marr BP, Shields CL, Zeolite I, Abramson DH. Extraocular extension of uveal melanoma after fine-needle aspiration, vitrectomy, and open biopsy. JAMA Ophthalmol. 2013;131(9):1220–4. https://doi.org/10.1001/jamaophthalmol.2013.2506.

19. Singh AD, Medina CA, Singh N, Aronow ME, Biscotti CV, Triozzi PL. Fine-needle aspiration biopsy of uveal melanoma: outcomes and complications. Br J Ophthalmol. 2016;100(4):456–62. https://doi.org/10.1136/bjophthalmol-2015-306921.

20. Shields CL, Ganguly A, Materin MA, Teixeira L, Mashayekhi A, Swanson LA, Marr BP, Shields JA. Chromosome 3 analysis of uveal melanoma using fine-needle aspiration biopsy at the time of plaque radiotherapy in 140 consecutive cases: the Deborah Iverson, MD, Lectureship. Arch Ophthalmol. 2007;125(8):1017–24. https://doi.org/10.1001/archopht.125.8.1017.

21. Correa ZM, Augsburger JJ. Sufficiency of FNAB aspirates of posterior uveal melanoma for cytologic versus GEP classification in 159 patients, and relative prognostic significance of these classifications. Graefes Arch Clin Exp Ophthalmol. 2014;252(1):131–5. https://doi.org/10.1007/s00417-013-2515-0.

22. Kim RS, Chevez-Barrios P, Divatia M, Bretana ME, Teh BS, Schefler AC. Transvitreal and transscleral biopsies in small uveal melanoma: report on yield, techniques, and complications. JAMA Ophthalmol. 2018;2(4):208–12.

23. Melia BM, Abramson DH, Albert DM, Boldt HC, Earle JD, Hanson WF, Montague P, Moy CS, Schachat AP, Simpson ER, Straatsma BR, Vine AK, Weingeist TA, Collaborative Ocular Melanoma Study Group. Collaborative ocular melanoma study (COMS) randomized trial of I-125 brachytherapy for medium choroidal melanoma. I. Visual acuity after 3 years COMS report no. 16. Ophthalmology. 2001;108(2):348–66.

24. American Brachytherapy Society–Ophthalmic Oncology Task Force. Electronic Address Pec, Committee AO. The American Brachytherapy Society consensus guidelines for plaque brachytherapy of uveal melanoma and retinoblastoma. Brachytherapy. 2014;13(1):1–14. https://doi.org/10.1016/j.brachy.2013.11.008.

25. Nag S, Quivey JM, Earle JD, Followill D, Fontanesi J, Finger PT, American Brachytherapy S. The American Brachytherapy Society recommendations for brachytherapy of uveal melanomas. Int J Radiat Oncol Biol Phys. 2003;56(2):544–55.

26. Astrahan MA, Luxton G, Pu Q, Petrovich Z. Conformal episcleral plaque therapy. Int J Radiat Oncol Biol Phys. 1997;39(2):505–19.

27. King B, Morales-Tirado VM, Wynn HG, Gao BT, Ballo MT, Wilson MW. Repeat episcleral plaque brachytherapy: clinical outcomes in patients treated for locally recurrent posterior uveal melanoma. Am J Ophthalmol. 2017;176:40–5. https://doi.org/10.1016/j.ajo.2016.12.022.

28. Aziz HA, Al Zahrani YA, Bena J, Lorek B, Wilkinson A, Suh J, Singh AD. Episcleral brachytherapy of uveal melanoma: role of intraoperative echographic confirmation. Br J Ophthalmol. 2017;101(6):747–51. https://doi.org/10.1136/bjophthalmol-2016-309153.

29. Tabandeh H, Chaudhry NA, Murray TG, Ehlies F, Hughes R, Scott IU, Markoe AM. Intraoperative echographic localization of iodine-125 episcleral plaque for brachytherapy of choroidal melanoma. Am J Ophthalmol. 2000;129(2):199–204.

30. Mruthyunjaya P, Seider MI, Stinnett S, Schefler A, Ocular Oncology Study Consortium. Association between tumor regression rate and gene expression profile after iodine 125 plaque radiotherapy for uveal melanoma. Ophthalmology. 2017;124(10):1532–9. https://doi.org/10.1016/j.ophtha.2017.04.013.

31. Ophthalmic Oncology Task Force. Local recurrence significantly increases the risk of metastatic uveal melanoma. Ophthalmology. 2016;123(1):86–91. https://doi.org/10.1016/j.ophtha.2015.09.014.

32. Force OOT. Local recurrence significantly increases the risk of metastatic uveal melanoma. Ophthalmology. 2016;123(1):86–91. https://doi.org/10.1016/j.ophtha.2015.09.014.

33. Collaborative Ocular Melanoma Study Group. The COMS randomized trial of iodine 125 brachytherapy for choroidal melanoma: V. Twelve-year mortality rates and prognostic factors: COMS report No. 28. Arch Ophthalmol. 2006;124(12):1684–93. https://doi.org/10.1001/archopht.124.12.1684.

34. Berry JL, Dandapani SV, Stevanovic M, Lee TC, Astrahan M, Murphree AL, Kim JW. Outcomes of choroidal melanomas treated with eye physics: a 20-year review. JAMA Ophthalmol. 2013;131(11):1435–42. https://doi.org/10.1001/jamaophthalmol.2013.4422.

35. Tann AW, Teh BS, Scarboro SB, Lewis GD, Bretana ME, Croft PC, Raizen Y, Butler EB, Kim RS, Chevez-Barrios P, Schefler AC. Early outcomes of uveal melanoma treated with intra-operative ultrasound guided brachytherapy using custom built plaques. Pract Radiat Oncol. 2017;7(4):e275–82. https://doi.org/10.1016/j.prro.2017.01.002.

36. McCannel TA, Chang MY, Burgess BL. Multi-year follow-up of fine-needle aspiration biopsy in choroidal melanoma. Ophthalmology. 2012;119(3):606–10. https://doi.org/10.1016/j.ophtha.2011.08.046.

37. Seibel I, Cordini D, Rehak M, Hager A, Riechardt AI, Boker A, Heufelder J, Weber A, Gollrad J, Besserer A, Joussen AM. Local recurrence after primary proton beam therapy in uveal mela-noma: risk factors, retreatment approaches, and outcome. Am J Ophthalmol. 2015;160(4):628–36. https://doi.org/10.1016/j.ajo.2015.06.017.

38. Desjardins L, Lumbroso L, Levy C, Mazal A, Delacroix S, Rosenwald JC, Dendale R, Plancher C, Asselain B. Treatment of uveal melanoma with iodine 125 plaques or proton beam therapy: indications and comparison of local recurrence rates. J Fr Ophthalmol. 2003;26(3):269–76.

39. Pereira PR, Odashiro AN, Lim LA, Miyamoto C, Blanco PL, Odashiro M, Maloney S, De Souza DF, Burnier MN Jr. Current and emerging treatment options for uveal melanoma. Clin Ophthalmol. 2013;7:1669–82. https://doi.org/10.2147/OPTH.S28863.

40. Finger PT, Chin KJ, Semenova EA. Intravitreal anti-VEGF therapy for macular radiation retinopathy: a 10-year study. Eur J Ophthalmol. 2016;26(1):60–6. https://doi.org/10.5301/ejo.5000670.

41. Mashayekhi A, Rojanaporn D, Al-Dahmash S, Shields CL, Shields JA. Monthly intravitreal bevacizumab for macular edema after iodine-125 plaque radiotherapy of uveal melanoma. Eur J Ophthalmol. 2014;24(2):228–34. https://doi.org/10.5301/ejo.5000352.

42. Kim IK, Lane AM, Jain P, Awh C, Gragoudas ES. Ranibizumab for the prevention of radiation complications in patients treated with proton beam irradiation for choroidal melanoma. Trans Am Ophthalmol Soc. 2016;114:T2.

43. Komatsubara KM, Carvajal RD. Immunotherapy for the treatment of uveal melanoma: cur-rent status and emerging therapies. Curr Oncol Rep. 2017;19(7):45. https://doi.org/10.1007/s11912-017-0606-5.

44. Triozzi PL, Singh AD. Adjuvant therapy of uveal melanoma: current status. Ocul Oncol Pathol. 2014;1(1):54–62. https://doi.org/10.1159/000367715.

45. Lane AM, Egan KM, Harmon D, Holbrook A, Munzenrider JE, Gragoudas ES. Adjuvant inter-feron therapy for patients with uveal melanoma at high risk of metastasis. Ophthalmology. 2009;116(11):2206–12. https://doi.org/10.1016/j.ophtha.2009.04.044.

46. Jager MJ, Dogrusoz M, Woodman SE. Uveal melanoma: identifying immunological and che-motherapeutic targets to treat metastases. Asia Pac J Ophthalmol. 2017;6(2):179–85. https://doi.org/10.22608/APO.201782.

47. Luke JJ, Callahan MK, Postow MA, Romano E, Ramaiya N, Bluth M, Giobbie-Hurder A, Lawrence DP, Ibrahim N, Ott PA, Flaherty KT, Sullivan RJ, Harding JJ, D'Angelo S, Dickson M, Schwartz GK, Chapman PB, Wolchok JD, Hodi FS, Carvajal RD. Clinical activity of ipi-limumab for metastatic uveal melanoma: a retrospective review of the Dana-Farber Cancer Institute, Massachusetts General Hospital, Memorial Sloan-Kettering Cancer Center, and University Hospital of Lausanne experience. Cancer. 2013;119(20):3687–95. https://doi.org/10.1002/cncr.28282.

48. Algazi AP, Tsai KK, Shoushtari AN, Munhoz RR, Eroglu Z, Piulats JM, Ott PA, Johnson DB, Hwang J, Daud AI, Sosman JA, Carvajal RD, Chmielowski B, Postow MA, Weber JS, Sullivan RJ. Clinical outcomes in metastatic uveal melanoma treated with PD-1 and PD-L1 antibodies. Cancer. 2016;122(21):3344–53. https://doi.org/10.1002/cncr.30258.

49. Field MG, Decatur CL, Kurtenbach S, Gezgin G, van der Velden PA, Jager MJ, Kozak KN, Harbour JW. PRAME as an independent biomarker for metastasis in uveal melanoma. Clin Cancer Res. 2016;22(5):1234–42. https://doi.org/10.1158/1078-0432.CCR-15-2071.

50. Gezgin G, Luk SJ, Cao J, Dogrusoz M, van der Steen DM, Hagedoorn RS, Krijgsman D, van der Velden PA, Field MG, Luyten GPM, Szuhai K, Harbour JW, Jordanova ES, Heemskerk MHM, Jager MJ. PRAME as a potential target for immunotherapy in metastatic uveal melanoma. JAMA Ophthalmol. 2017;135(6):541–9. https://doi.org/10.1001/jamaophthalmol.2017.0729.
51. Kines RC, Varsavsky I, Choudhary S, Bhattacharya D, Spring S, McLaughlin RJ, Kang SJ, Grossniklaus HE, Vavvas DG, Monks S, MacDougall JR, de Los Pinos E, Schiller JT. An infrared dye-conjugated virus-like particle for the treatment of primary uveal melanoma. Mol Cancer Ther. 2018;17(2):565–74. https://doi.org/10.1158/1535-7163.MCT-17-0953.

Genetic Implications of Ocular Melanoma

Mona Mohammad and Mandeep S. Sagoo

Introduction

The management of uveal melanoma (UM) has steadily improved over the last century. The majority of eyes with UM can now be salvaged with radiotherapy, most commonly with plaque radiotherapy or proton beam radiotherapy. Tumors beyond the scope of radiotherapy still necessitate enucleation. Despite the improvement in the therapeutic options for UM, up to half of all patients will develop metastasis irrespective of the primary treatment given [1–3]. Mortality has not improved over the last 30 years, and many centers now offer treatment earlier in order to improve systemic prognosis [4]. UMs metastasize by hematogenous dissemination, and the most common sites of metastasis are liver (93%), lung (24%), and bone (16%).The survival for these patients is poor since UM is resistant to standard treatments with systemic chemotherapy [5, 6].

Given the high risk for metastasis and the poor life expectancy thereafter, identifying high-risk features for metastasis at the time of diagnosis of UM is important for both patients and physicians because it allows for earlier detection of metastasis, personalized clinical decision-making, and the hope that more targeted therapeutic options will be offered for high-risk patients.

Traditionally, clinicopathological features of UMs were used to provide an estimation of the metastatic risk. Those having older patient age, larger tumor basal

M. Mohammad
Ocular Oncology Service, Moorfields Eye Hospital, London, UK
e-mail: mona.mohammad@moorfields.nhs.uk

M. S. Sagoo (✉)
Ocular Oncology Service, Moorfields Eye Hospital, London, UK

NIHR Biomedical Research Centre for Ophthalmology at Moorfields Eye Hospital
and UCL Institute of Ophthalmology, London, UK
e-mail: mandeep.sagoo@nhs.net

© Springer Nature Singapore Pte Ltd. 2019
A. Ramasubramanian (ed.), *Ocular Oncology*, Current Practices in
Ophthalmology, https://doi.org/10.1007/978-981-13-7538-5_3

diameter, invasion of the sclera, ciliary body involvement, and epithelioid cell type have been associated with worse final prognosis and a higher incidence of metastatic disease [7, 8].

Recently, with rapid development of new molecular techniques, the understanding of the genetic makeup of tumor cells has improved, leading to more accurate prognostic information becoming available [9–12].

Methods of Genetic Testing

The ocular oncologist needs to establish a collaboration with a molecular genetics laboratory in order to undertake genetic analysis of harvested cells. This can be achieved through a research facility, a local specialist diagnostic genetics laboratory, or commercial arrangements.

Patient consent should be obtained for genetic testing of the tumor cells. In many centers diagnostic genetic testing is now the standard of care in UM management but in some centers it remains a research tool and hence ethical approval may be required. The consent process begins during the patient consultation when the melanoma is diagnosed. The risks and benefits of testing should be discussed with the patient in the light of the primary treatment. For example, in enucleation cases the harvesting of tumor cells once the eye is removed poses no physical risk to the patient but in eyes being treated by conservative means a fine-needle aspirate (FNAB) is required which may pose risks such as hemorrhage, reduced vision, and tumor seeding. A mutual decision between the patient and the surgeon is taken. Variations exist in practice amongst ocular oncologists as to the utility of routine performance of FNAB for cytogenetics. It can be argued that there is little advantage in undertaking this step, as it does not routinely alter therapy of micrometastatic disease due to the paucity of adjuvant treatments currently available. On the contrary, it can be useful for the patient and their physician to have a more accurate idea of prognosis to inform the frequency of systemic screening investigations. The patient should also be made aware of insufficient diagnostic yield, though insufficient diagnostic yield may reflect biological cohesiveness of the tumor and hence a lower propensity for metastatic disease [13].

A small quantity of fresh tumor cells is extracted from the tumor. This can be by punch biopsy or FNAB after enucleation or it can be by FNAB at the time of radioactive plaque insertion or insertion of tantalum marker clips in preparation for proton beam radiotherapy. Tissue samples can also be obtained from an enucleation specimen that has been formalin-fixed and paraffin-embedded (FFPE), but many laboratories find diagnostic quality poor.

Studies comparing trans-scleral with vitrectomy-assisted transvitreal fine-needle aspiration biopsy found similar tissue yield for both techniques for subsequent cytopathologic analysis [14].

Samples are then sent for DNA extraction that can allow for further analysis of the tumor through different genetic studies: karyotyping, fluorescence in situ hybridization (FISH), comparative genomic hybridization (CGH), multiplex ligation-dependent probe amplification (MLPA), or gene expression profiling (GEP) [15]. Chromosomal and gene defects have been implicated in UM.

Genetic Abnormalities in UM

Chromosome 3

In 1990, Prescher et al. studied chromosomal abnormalities in UM. They reported that monosomy 3 (complete loss of one copy of chromosome 3) and increased copies of the long arm of chromosome 8q (+8q) were commonly found in UM samples [16]. These findings opened the doors for further studies to look into the prognostic implications of monosomy 3 in UM; and later it was found that monosomy 3 is associated with other clinicopathological factors (larger tumor diameter, ciliary body involvement, epithelioid cells, and closed loops) that are known to be related to aggressive tumor behavior [11, 17, 18].

Other forms of chromosome 3 abnormalities have been observed in UM; these include partial deletions in the short (3p) or long (3q) arms and minor abnormalities affecting localized regions of chromosome 3 [19]. Isodisomy 3 (acquired homozygosity) where both chromosomes are from the same parent is prognostically equivalent to monosomy 3 and has also been linked to UM [20].

Chromosome 8

Chromosome 8 abnormalities are also associated with UM; tumors with additional copies of 8q have also been linked with poor survival prognosis [10]. Chromosome 8q gain most commonly coexists with monosomy 3, and tumors having both mutations are associated with poor prognosis than those having 8q gain alone or monosomy 3 alone [21].

Chromosome 6

In contrast to changes in chromosomes 3 and 8, chromosome 6 gain is a strong indicator of good prognosis of UM, and has an inverse relationship with the risk of melanoma metastasis [9, 22].

Chromosome 1

Chromosome 1p loss is another poor prognostic factor in UM; the risk of melanoma metastasis is increased for tumors with monosomy 3 and chromosome 1p loss [23].

Class 1/Class 2 UM

Gene expression profiling (GEP), also known as transcriptomics, uses microarrays to simultaneously compare gene transcription (in thousands of genes) between normal and cancer cells. GEP allows for the identification of genes that are overexpressed or underexpressed in tumor cells. By applying GEP on UM, two distinct classes were found:

- Class 1 tumors (all cells have disomy 3) are low-grade tumors and a lower risk of metastasis.
- Class 2 tumors (all cells have monosomy 3) are high-grade tumors with an increased tendency to metastasize [24, 25].

Class 1 tumor cells closely resemble normal uveal melanocytes and low-grade, differentiated uveal melanocytic tumors, whereas class 2 tumor cells resemble primitive undifferentiated neural/ectodermal cells [26, 27].

Currently, gene expression profiling is superior to all of the known factors at predicting metastatic spread of the primary UM, including monosomy 3 [28]. The latest TNM edition encourages recording of genetic profile for these tumors [29].

The importance of clinical factors cannot be overlooked and the interpretation of cytogenetic testing must take other clinical and pathological data into consideration. In class 2 UM, prognosis is better when largest basal diameter is less than 12 mm; this shows the importance of appropriate management of the primary melanoma as soon as possible [30, 31].

When performing GEP from a single tumor site, one should keep in mind that there is a risk of misclassification, due to tumor heterogeneity. It was noted that this heterogeneity is more obvious for small tumors [32].

DecisionDx-UM is a prognostic test that assesses GEP of tumor cells and then classifies tumors into three different classes: class 1A (low metastatic risk), class 1B (long-term metastatic risk), or class 2 (immediate, high metastatic risk). The 5-year metastatic risk is 2%, 21%, and 72% for class 1A, 1B, and 2, respectively [33].

Mutational Profiling in UM: Towards Pathogenesis

While chromosomal abnormalities help in prognostication of patients with UM, detection of specific mutations in UM may provide in addition new insights into the pathogenesis of this tumor, in the hope that targets specifically against these mutations lead to improved therapeutic options with novel drugs.

The genetic profile of UM differs from cutaneous melanoma (CM). The number of mutations identified so far for UM is less than that found in CM. For example, UM lacks mutations often found in CM such as in BRAF, NRAS, or KIT. A different set of genes with oncogenic or loss-of-function mutations appear to be implicated in UM, adding to the notion that UM is a biologically distinct entity to CM [34–37]. Germline mutation in the CDKN2A gene is the strongest known inherited risk factor for CM, but having these mutations does not increase the risk of UM [38, 39].

GNAQ and GNA11 Gene Mutations

Gαq and Gα11 are two closely related G-coupled protein receptor (Gq) alpha subunits. The genes for these proteins are GNAQ (Chr. 9q21.2) and GNA11 (Chr19p13.3), respectively.

GNAQ gene was found to be mutated in 49% of UMs. In fact, GNAQ mutation represents the most common known oncogenic mutation in this tumor. This mutation represents an early or initiating event, found in tumors at all stages of malignant progression, and this explains why GNAQ mutation is not associated with any clinical, pathologic, or molecular features associated with late tumor progression [40]. GNAQ mutations were also discovered in 83% of blue nevi of the skin [41]. GNA11 gene mutations were found in 32% of UM samples and 57% of UM metastases.

Mutations in GNAQ and GNA11 affect a critical oncogenic signaling cascade that affects the metastatic potential of tumors [42]. These mutations (GNAQ and GNA11) are mutually exclusive and represent early or initiating events that constitutively activate the mitogen-activated protein kinase (MAPK) pathway and play an essential role in the development of UMs [41, 43].

Although identifying GNAQ mutation status does not predict tumor progression, the high frequency of these mutations may render it a promising target for therapeutic intervention [44].

BRCA1-Associated Protein 1 (BAP1) Gene Mutations

BRCA1-associated protein 1 (BAP1) gene, located at chromosome 3p21, is a tumor-suppressor and metastasis-suppressor gene. BAP1 gene encodes a protein with a ubiquitin carboxy-terminal hydrolase (UCH) domain that gives BAP1 its deubiquitinase activity.

In 2010, Harbour et al. identified inactivating mutations in BAP1 in 47% of UMs. Their group was also the first to show germline BAP1 mutations, and that BAP1 mutation was strongly associated with metastasis. This study also identified a germline mutation in one of the UM patients, suggesting that, besides being a metastasis suppressor, BAP1 could predispose certain people to more aggressive UM tumors [45].

Whereas BAP1 mutations are rare in class 1 tumors, they are found in approximately 85% of class 2 UMs, suggesting that BAP1 may function as a metastasis suppressor in this cancer [46, 47].

BAP1-Tumor Predisposition Syndrome (BAP1-TPDS)

UM is a sporadic disease, but cases of familial UM have been reported. These patients present at an early age and tend to have more aggressive tumors [48]. The only high-penetrance susceptibility gene for familial UM identified so far is the BAP1 gene. The cancer risk mediated by germline BAP1 mutations is inherited in an autosomal dominant (AD) pattern with incomplete penetrance. Patients with germline BAP1 mutations are at risk of developing several other cancers (cutaneous melanoma (CM), renal cell carcinoma (RCC), basal cell carcinoma, meningioma, malignant mesothelioma (MM) with UM being the most common tumor in BAP1-TPDS). The risk of having UM in germline BAP1 mutation carriers is 29% [49, 50].

Patients with early-onset UM (age <30 years), multifocal UM, or personal or family history of two or more of UM, RCC, MM, and CM should be suspected of having germline BAP1 mutations. These patients are managed as high-risk patients and should be monitored accordingly [51, 52].

Splicing Factor 3B Subunit 1 (SF3B1) Mutations

This gene, located at Ch. 2q33.1, encodes subunit 1 of the splicing factor 3b protein complex. SF3B1 mutations are largely mutually exclusive with BAP1 mutations and are associated with favorable prognosis [53–55].

Eukaryotic Translation Initiation Factor (EIF1AX)

Mutations in this X-chromosome gene that encodes for eIF1AX- protein were found in tumors with disomy 3 [56]. EIF1AX-mutated tumors show strong correlation with class 1 GEP tumors and improvement in patient survival [52].

In summary, GNAQ, GNA11, BAP1, SF3B1, and EIF1AX gene mutations are commonly seen in UM; GNAQ and GNA11 are mutually exclusive, occur early, and do not have prognostic values. BAP1, SF3B1, and EIFAX are also mutually exclusive, occur late, and are prognostically significant (poor prognosis for BAP1, while SF3B1 and EIF1AX have favorable prognosis) [57].

Advantages and Disadvantages of Genetic Testing

Knowing the specific genetic alterations in UM will allow us to identify those at higher risk of systemic involvement. This information can help decide their future plans as well as the argument that they should be given more intensive follow-up screening protocols to detect metastasis at early stages. In the future, once therapy becomes available for micrometastatic disease, this is the group that targeted therapy will be most useful for, hence prolonging overall survival and improving the quality of life.

The Limitations of Genetic Testing

- The sample has to be taken from the tumor, that is, there is no blood marker yet.
- May not be reliable after radiation treatment due to alteration of DNA and/or RNA of tumor cells.
- Tumor heterogeneity where performing biopsy sample from a single tumor site carries a risk of prognostic misclassification—a risk in smaller tumors.
- Insufficient samples and thus the need for larger tissue biopsy.
- Procedure-specific risks, including hemorrhage, retinal detachment, or tumor seeding.
- Not available in all centers in the world.
- Psychological effects of being in a high-risk genetic profile group.

Therapy

Despite excellent local tumor control of UM, metastasis is high. Treatment options are limited with poor life expectancy [58]. With emerging understanding of the molecular events in UM, more clinical trials will elicit the use of targeted novel therapies, namely kinase inhibitors and immunotherapy for selected patients [59–61].

As stated previously, mutations in G protein alpha subunit q and 11 (GNAQ/11) are common early events in UM patients, with subsequent production of abnormal proteins that activate the MAP kinase pathway. Given the early occurrence of GNAQ/11 mutations in UM it is not optimal to target these mutations. Also there are no clinically available specific inhibitors of GNAQ/11.

An alternative therapeutic strategy is the targeting of downstream effectors MAPK kinase enzyme (MEK). Of particular interest is selumetinib which is an orally administered drug that blocks the enzyme MAPK kinase (MEK) and thus disrupts the MEK pathway. This drug was found to inhibit the growth of GNAQ-mutated UM cell lines [62, 63]. Moreover, selumetinib has also been shown to play a role in tumor shrinkage [64].

A randomized phase II trial for patients with metastatic UM showed better progression-free survival (PFS) with selumetinib monotherapy (median 15.9 weeks) versus chemotherapy with temozolomide or dacarbazine (median 7 weeks); tumor regression was observed in 49% of patients treated with selumetinib [65].

Conclusion

UM is the most common primary intraocular malignancy in adults. Treatment of this tumor gives excellent local tumor control, but metastasis remains a challenge. There is no effective treatment for metastatic UM. Several approaches are necessary to improve systemic prognosis: early treatment of the primary tumor, development of effective adjuvant treatments in high-risk patients, and better therapy for established metastatic involvement. Early diagnosis at a time when the tumor is small and at least risk for metastatic disease is currently the best way to decrease mortality. Various clinical, histopathological, cytogenetics, and molecular markers are used to predict prognosis and to identify patients with high risk for metastasis. The molecular pathways involved in UM are only just being elucidated. This effort will yield targets to harness in order to improve survival.

References

1. Singh AD, Turell ME, Topham AK. Uveal melanoma: trends in incidence, treatment, and survival. Ophthalmology. 2011;118(9):1881–5.
2. Virgili G, et al. Survival in patients with uveal melanoma in Europe. Arch Ophthalmol. 2008;126(10):1413–8.
3. Collaborative Ocular Melanoma Study Group. The COMS randomized trial of iodine 125 brachytherapy for choroidal melanoma: V. Twelve-year mortality rates and prognostic factors: COMS report No. 28. Arch Ophthalmol. 2006;124(12):1684–93.
4. Vasalaki M, et al. Ocular oncology: advances in retinoblastoma, uveal melanoma and conjunctival melanoma. Br Med Bull. 2017;121(1):107–19.
5. Collaborative Ocular Melanoma Study Group. Assessment of metastatic disease status at death in 435 patients with large choroidal melanoma in the Collaborative Ocular Melanoma Study (COMS): COMS report no. 15. Arch Ophthalmol. 2001;119(5):670–6.
6. Diener-West M, et al. Development of metastatic disease after enrollment in the COMS trials for treatment of choroidal melanoma: Collaborative Ocular Melanoma Study Group report no. 26. Arch Ophthalmol. 2005;123(12):1639–43.
7. McLean IW, Foster WD, Zimmerman LE. Uveal melanoma: location, size, cell type, and enucleation as risk factors in metastasis. Hum Pathol. 1982;13(2):123–32.
8. Al-Jamal RT, Makitie T, Kivela T. Nucleolar diameter and microvascular factors as independent predictors of mortality from malignant melanoma of the choroid and ciliary body. Invest Ophthalmol Vis Sci. 2003;44(6):2381–9.
9. White VA, et al. Correlation of cytogenetic abnormalities with the outcome of patients with uveal melanoma. Cancer. 1998;83(2):354–9.
10. Sisley K, et al. Abnormalities of chromosomes 3 and 8 in posterior uveal melanoma correlate with prognosis. Genes Chromosomes Cancer. 1997;19(1):22–8.
11. Scholes AG, et al. Monosomy 3 in uveal melanoma: correlation with clinical and histologic predictors of survival. Invest Ophthalmol Vis Sci. 2003;44(3):1008–11.
12. Kaliki S, Shields CL, Shields JA. Uveal melanoma: estimating prognosis. Indian J Ophthalmol. 2015;63(2):93–102.
13. Augsburger JJ, Correa ZM, Trichopoulos N. Prognostic implications of cytopathologic classification of melanocytic uveal tumors evaluated by fine-needle aspiration biopsy. Arq Bras Oftalmol. 2013;76(2):72–9.
14. Chang MY, McCannel TA. Comparison of uveal melanoma cytopathologic sample retrieval in trans-scleral versus vitrectomy-assisted transvitreal fine needle aspiration biopsy. Br J Ophthalmol. 2014;98(12):1654–8.
15. Schopper VJ, Correa ZM. Clinical application of genetic testing for posterior uveal melanoma. Int J Retina Vitreous. 2016;2:4.
16. Prescher G, Bornfeld N, Becher R. Nonrandom chromosomal abnormalities in primary uveal melanoma. J Natl Cancer Inst. 1990;82(22):1765–9.
17. Patel KA, et al. Prediction of prognosis in patients with uveal melanoma using fluorescence in situ hybridisation. Br J Ophthalmol. 2001;85(12):1440–4.
18. Shields CL, et al. Personalized prognosis of uveal melanoma based on cytogenetic profile in 1059 patients over an 8-year period: the 2017 Harry S. Gradle lecture. Ophthalmology. 2017;124(10):1523–31.

19. Tschentscher F, et al. Partial deletions of the long and short arm of chromosome 3 point to two tumor suppressor genes in uveal melanoma. Cancer Res. 2001;61(8):3439–42.
20. White VA, McNeil BK, Horsman DE. Acquired homozygosity (isodisomy) of chromosome 3 in uveal melanoma. Cancer Genet Cytogenet. 1998;102(1):40–5.
21. Aalto Y, et al. Concomitant loss of chromosome 3 and whole arm losses and gains of chromosome 1, 6, or 8 in metastasizing primary uveal melanoma. Invest Ophthalmol Vis Sci. 2001;42(2):313–7.
22. Damato B, et al. Multiplex ligation-dependent probe amplification of uveal melanoma: correlation with metastatic death. Invest Ophthalmol Vis Sci. 2009;50(7):3048–55.
23. Kilic E, et al. Concurrent loss of chromosome arm 1p and chromosome 3 predicts a decreased disease-free survival in uveal melanoma patients. Invest Ophthalmol Vis Sci. 2005;46(7):2253–7.
24. Tschentscher F, et al. Tumor classification based on gene expression profiling shows that uveal melanomas with and without monosomy 3 represent two distinct entities. Cancer Res. 2003;63(10):2578–84.
25. Onken MD, et al. Gene expression profiling in uveal melanoma reveals two molecular classes and predicts metastatic death. Cancer Res. 2004;64(20):7205–9.
26. Onken MD, et al. Functional gene expression analysis uncovers phenotypic switch in aggressive uveal melanomas. Cancer Res. 2006;66(9):4602–9.
27. Chang SH, et al. Prognostic biomarkers in uveal melanoma: evidence for a stem cell-like phenotype associated with metastasis. Melanoma Res. 2008;18(3):191–200.
28. Kivela T, Kujala E. Prognostication in eye cancer: the latest tumor, node, metastasis classification and beyond. Eye (Lond). 2013;27(2):243–52.
29. Edge SB, Compton CC. The American Joint Committee on Cancer: the 7th edition of the AJCC cancer staging manual and the future of TNM. Ann Surg Oncol. 2010;17(6):1471–4.
30. Walter SD, et al. Prognostic implications of tumor diameter in association with gene expression profile for uveal melanoma. JAMA Ophthalmol. 2016;134(7):734–40.
31. Damato B, et al. Cytogenetics of uveal melanoma: a 7-year clinical experience. Ophthalmology. 2007;114(10):1925–31.
32. Augsburger JJ, Correa ZM, Augsburger BD. Frequency and implications of discordant gene expression profile class in posterior uveal melanomas sampled by fine needle aspiration biopsy. Am J Ophthalmol. 2015;159(2):248–56.
33. Field MG, Harbour JW. Recent developments in prognostic and predictive testing in uveal melanoma. Curr Opin Ophthalmol. 2014;25(3):234–9.
34. Saldanha G, et al. High BRAF mutation frequency does not characterize all melanocytic tumor types. Int J Cancer. 2004;111(5):705–10.
35. Zuidervaart W, et al. Activation of the MAPK pathway is a common event in uveal melanomas although it rarely occurs through mutation of BRAF or RAS. Br J Cancer. 2005;92(11):2032–8.
36. Fecher LA, et al. Toward a molecular classification of melanoma. J Clin Oncol. 2007;25(12):1606–20.
37. van den Bosch T, et al. Genetics of uveal melanoma and cutaneous melanoma: two of a kind? Dermatol Res Pract. 2010;2010:360136.
38. Davies H, et al. Mutations of the BRAF gene in human cancer. Nature. 2002;417(6892):949–54.
39. Pollock PM, et al. High frequency of BRAF mutations in nevi. Nat Genet. 2003;33(1):19–20.
40. Onken MD, et al. Oncogenic mutations in GNAQ occur early in uveal melanoma. Invest Ophthalmol Vis Sci. 2008;49(12):5230–4.
41. Van Raamsdonk CD, et al. Frequent somatic mutations of GNAQ in uveal melanoma and blue naevi. Nature. 2009;457(7229):599–602.
42. Van Raamsdonk CD, et al. Mutations in GNA11 in uveal melanoma. N Engl J Med. 2010;363(23):2191–9.
43. Wan PT, et al. Mechanism of activation of the RAF-ERK signaling pathway by oncogenic mutations of B-RAF. Cell. 2004;116(6):855–67.
44. Bauer J, et al. Oncogenic GNAQ mutations are not correlated with disease-free survival in uveal melanoma. Br J Cancer. 2009;101(5):813–5.

45. Harbour JW, et al. Frequent mutation of BAP1 in metastasizing uveal melanomas. Science. 2010;330(6009):1410–3.
46. Jensen DE, et al. BAP1: a novel ubiquitin hydrolase which binds to the BRCA1 RING finger and enhances BRCA1-mediated cell growth suppression. Oncogene. 1998;16(9):1097–112.
47. Dey A, et al. Loss of the tumor suppressor BAP1 causes myeloid transformation. Science. 2012;337(6101):1541–6.
48. Gupta MP, et al. Clinical characteristics of uveal melanoma in patients with germline BAP1 mutations. JAMA Ophthalmol. 2015;133(8):881–7.
49. Rai K, et al. Comprehensive review of BAP1 tumor predisposition syndrome with report of two new cases. Clin Genet. 2016;89(3):285–94.
50. Rednam KR, et al. Uveal melanoma in association with multiple malignancies. A case report and review. Retina. 1981;1(2):100–6.
51. Masoomian B, Shields JA, Shields CL. Overview of BAP1 cancer predisposition syndrome and the relationship to uveal melanoma. J Curr Ophthalmol. 2018;30(2):102–9.
52. Helgadottir H, Hoiom V. The genetics of uveal melanoma: current insights. Appl Clin Genet. 2016;9:147–55.
53. Papaemmanuil E, et al. Somatic SF3B1 mutation in myelodysplasia with ring sideroblasts. N Engl J Med. 2011;365(15):1384–95.
54. Wang L, et al. SF3B1 and other novel cancer genes in chronic lymphocytic leukemia. N Engl J Med. 2011;365(26):2497–506.
55. Yavuzyigitoglu S, et al. Uveal melanomas with SF3B1 mutations: a distinct subclass associated with late-onset metastases. Ophthalmology. 2016;123(5):1118–28.
56. Martin M, et al. Exome sequencing identifies recurrent somatic mutations in EIF1AX and SF3B1 in uveal melanoma with disomy 3. Nat Genet. 2013;45(8):933–6.
57. Decatur CL, et al. Driver mutations in uveal melanoma: associations with gene expression profile and patient outcomes. JAMA Ophthalmol. 2016;134(7):728–33.
58. Augsburger JJ, Correa ZM, Shaikh AH. Effectiveness of treatments for metastatic uveal melanoma. Am J Ophthalmol. 2009;148(1):119–27.
59. Patel M, et al. Therapeutic implications of the emerging molecular biology of uveal melanoma. Clin Cancer Res. 2011;17(8):2087–100.
60. Sagoo MS, et al. Combined PKC and MEK inhibition for treating metastatic uveal melanoma. Oncogene. 2014;33(39):4722–3.
61. Amirouchene-Angelozzi N, et al. Upcoming translational challenges for uveal melanoma. Br J Cancer. 2015;113(12):1746.
62. Ambrosini G, et al. Identification of unique MEK-dependent genes in GNAQ mutant uveal melanoma involved in cell growth, tumor cell invasion, and MEK resistance. Clin Cancer Res. 2012;18(13):3552–61.
63. Selumetinib shows promise in metastatic uveal melanoma. Cancer Discov. 2013;3(7):OF8.
64. Carvajal RD. et al. Pharmacodynamic activity of selumetinib to predict radiographic response in advanced uveal melanoma. American Society of Clinical Oncology; 2012.
65. Carvajal RD, et al. Effect of selumetinib vs. chemotherapy on progression-free survival in uveal melanoma: a randomized clinical trial. JAMA. 2014;311(23):2397–405.

Advancements in the Management of Optic Pathway Gliomas

Sahas Narain, Ashwini Kini, and Aparna Ramasubramanian

Introduction

Optic pathway gliomas account for about 1% of all intracranial tumors [1]. These tumors are pilocytic astrocyte tumors that can occur sporadically or due to neurofibromatosis type I (NF-1). Ninety percent of optic pathway tumors are either benign childhood gliomas or optic nerve sheath meningiomas; adult malignant gliomas are especially rare [2]. Most glioma cases occur in children under the age of 20. A younger age of onset generally correlates with poorer outcomes whereas NF-1-related optic nerve gliomas have better outcomes.

Optic pathway gliomas can sometimes be asymptomatic. Patients with NF-1 are more commonly asymptomatic compared to those with spontaneous gliomas [3]. When they do occur, symptoms are generally progressive due to slow enlargement of the tumor leading to proptosis and eventually displacement of the globe as the tumor expands. Decreased visual acuity can be an accompanying symptom along with decreased visual fields, RAPD, and disc swelling. Rarely, nystagmus could be a presenting symptom in children with chiasma/hypothalamus involving tumors [4]. Posterior optic nerve gliomas can also present as obstructive hydrocephalus or endocrinopathies. Precocious puberty is the most common hormonal disturbance from an optic glioma endocrinopathy [5, 6]. Other endocrinopathies that have been associated with OPG include growth hormone deficiency, obesity with insulin resistance/impaired glucose tolerance, GH excess, ACTH deficiency, hypogonadotropic

S. Narain
University of Louisville School of Medicine, Louisville, KY, USA
e-mail: smnara02@louisville.edu

A. Kini · A. Ramasubramanian (✉)
Department of Ophthalmology and Visual Sciences, University of Louisville, Louisville, KY, USA
e-mail: aparna.ramasubramanian@louisville.edu

© Springer Nature Singapore Pte Ltd. 2019
A. Ramasubramanian (ed.), *Ocular Oncology*, Current Practices in Ophthalmology, https://doi.org/10.1007/978-981-13-7538-5_4

hypogonadism, and thyrotropin deficiency [6]. Acute vision loss is a very rare complication that occurs when there is a hemorrhage in a tumor.

Severity of the tumor generally depends on the location of the tumor and can be divided into anterior visual pathway tumors and posterior visual pathway tumors. Posterior visual pathway tumors can be more aggressive and are generally more severe because the tumor can compress the chiasm and the hypothalamus (Fig. 1). These are more commonly associated with a sporadic tumor leading to more symptomatic presentations compared to those with NF-1, which are more commonly anterior visual pathway tumors [3]. Studies have demonstrated that the risk of vision loss is higher in more posteriorly located tumors and in older individuals and hence it is recommended that children with posteriorly located tumors have a close follow-up and visual assessment till the age of 18 [1]. A vast majority of these tumors pathologically fall under the category of pilocytic astrocytomas with a benign outcome. However, a small proportion of these tumors could run a more aggressive course, known as diffuse non-pilocytic astrocytomas. Spontaneous regression of clinically symptomatic tumor, both in patients with and without NF 1, has been reported in literature and could be associated with variable degree of visual improvement. This is a factor that should be considered while planning management of these tumors [7].

Diagnosis of optic nerve gliomas is confirmed by MRI. MRI is considered the best imaging due to its ability to show the entire path of the optic nerve to the hypothalamus to ensure that there is no hypothalamic involvement.

Chemo- and radiation treatment options have been successful in preventing severe visual disturbances by halting the progression of tumor growth. This chapter discusses the advancements in screening and treatment of optic nerve gliomas.

Fig. 1 Optic chiasmal glioma imaged with MRI

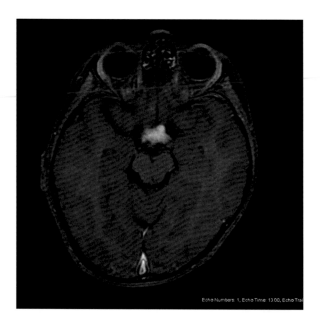

Screening

Current recommendations for screening children suggest that all children with NF1 younger than 8 years should undergo an annual ophthalmological examination that should include measurement of visual acuity, confrontation visual field evaluation, color vision testing, and assessment of pupils, eyelids, ocular motility, irises, and fundi (Table 1) [8]. Formal computerized or kinetic testing of visual fields may be adjunctive if the patient is reliable, but is not necessary.

Guidelines for evaluation of children under 1 year of age are not very clear; however Liu et al. recommend neuroimaging in this age group if the diagnosis is confirmed and visual assessment is unreliable to guide management.

Once children grow past the age of 8, the risk of development of OPG significantly decreases and there are no firm guidelines for follow-up protocol in this subset of children. Until new evidence is discovered, it is recommended that children in this age group should receive complete eye examinations every 2 years until they become 18 years old. After the age of 18, adults may have routine eye assessments without the need for specialized testing or imaging. Assessing color vision during an examination is also important because the presence of a visual acuity defect in the absence of a color vision defect would suggest other causes of an abnormal exam such as refractive error or amblyopia.

Visual evoked potential visual tests (VEP), though a sensitive method to detect optic nerve gliomas in asymptomatic children, is not routinely recommended. This is because it would not alter the management in the case of an asymptomatic patient. Even in symptomatic children with either low visual acuity, an abnormal fundus examination, or abnormal visual fields, neuroimaging is necessary regardless of the VEP report. Follow-up VEPs are also not recommended as subtle changes in the value are of uncertain significance and in the setting of stable visual and radiologic testing would not be a basis to start treatment [8].

Listernick et al. also recommended that the children have annual height and weight measurements to screen for precocious puberty [9]. This was further

Table 1 Screening protocol for optic nerve glioma

Screening	Frequency
Suspected or known NF1 with no OPG	Every year until age 8 years
	Every other year from 8 to 18 years
NF-1 OPG confirmed by MRI	Every 3 months for first year
Ophthalmology screening	Every 6 months for 2–8 years
	Annually from 8 to 18 years
NF-1 OPG confirmed by MRI	Every 3 months for first year
Neuroimaging	Every 6 months for 2 years
	Annually from 3 to 5 years
	Subsequently based on clinical judgement

Reproduced from de Blank PMK, Fisher MJ, Liu GT, Gutmann DH, Listernick R, Ferner RE, Avery RA. Optic pathway gliomas in neurofibromatosis type 1: an update: surveillance, treatment indications, and biomarkers of vision. J Neuroophthalmol. 2017;37(Suppl 1):S23–S32

confirmed by Segal et al. who reported a precocious puberty incidence of 14% in his retrospective chart review which followed 44 patients with OPG [10].

Risk for Progression

Using a multivariate analysis, Stokland et al. found factors that determine tumor progression in a childhood low-grade glioma including age, histology, and extent of resection. The risk of tumor progression decreases with age. A pathological diagnosis of fibrillary astrocytoma and pilomyxoid astrocytoma has poor outcomes in comparison to pilocytic astrocytoma. Finally, partial and incomplete surgical resection had poorer outcomes compared to complete tumor resection. They also found that the chiasmatic/hypothalamic group shows an early peak (4 years of age) and a declining incidence in subsequent age [10].

The possibility of sex playing a role in presentation was explored by Kelly et al. who found that females with NF1-associated optic gliomas were twice as likely to have undergone neuroimaging for visual symptoms and three times more likely than boys to require treatment due to visual decline, though the glioma location and size are not impacted by sex [11]. They further went on to explore the same in NF1 genetically engineered mice model and found that female mice were more likely than their male counterpart to have visual symptoms and were found to be associated with degeneration of retinal ganglion cells both in vivo and in vitro.

Imaging

Routine imaging for screening in NF1-positive patients is currently not recommended by AAP as the incidence and morbidity of these tumors are low. MRI is recommended only if symptoms such as visual changes, persistent headaches, or seizures occur as well as if there is a marked increase in head size or a plexiform neurofibroma of the head. A small percentage of the NF1 population that has a deletion of the entire NF1 gene with flanking DNA will also get a MRI [12]. CT scans do not have any advantage over MRIs and are not recommended for any imaging because they have additional risk of radiation exposure in children which can lead to secondary tumors.

Segal et al. discovered no additional benefit from routine baseline MRI imaging. The research group found that an earlier diagnosis did not end up having an effect on clinical outcome. Additionally, frequent imaging leads to repeated sedation and psychological effects on both the child and parents for a generally benign tumor that would require no further intervention. These adverse effects in addition to the financial burden of repeated imaging with no significant change in care support the idea of not requiring routine MRI [13].

The current protocol for imaging includes an MRI of the orbits and brain with thin, coronal, sagittal, and axial images both with and without contrast. It also includes both T1- and T2-weighted images with sections through the optic nerve.

OPGs have a typical appearance on MRI with fusiform enlargement and a downward kink in the mid orbit. Chiasmal tumors are better seen on coronal sections. Enhancement with gadolinium is a possible measure of activity in the tumor and could be used as a possible guide for treatment and follow-up (quote reference).

The tumor is typically hypointense on T1W images (Fig. 2c), and slightly hyperintense on T2W (Fig. 2d). Optic nerve gliomas (ONG) show increased diffusion on DWI; they exhibit high apparent diffusion coefficient (ADC) and low fractional anisotropy (FA) values. This is attributed to their low cellularity and low proliferative indices. ONGs show ADC values in the range of $1.2–2.09 \times 10^{-3}$ mm^2/s, which cannot however distinguish between clinically stable and aggressive tumors. In his cohort study, Yeom et al. found that a higher ADC predicted earlier tumor progression. However, there is insufficient data to include this in a routine protocol for imaging in OPG patients. They suggest that there is likely no benefit to treating a patient prior to onset of symptoms regardless of the ADC, but may prove to be useful in setting an appropriate clinical surveillance schedule and evaluating treatment responses [14].

DTI tractography can be used in the presurgical evaluation of ONG by demonstrating integrity of the optic nerve in patients with resectable lesions and can help reduce postsurgical morbidity and visual field loss [15].

De Blanc et al. suggest that in a MRI with diffusion tensor imaging (DTI), a decrease in FA (fractional anisotropy) of the optic radiations is associated with abnormal visual acuity in NF1-associated OPGs and may be predictive of visual

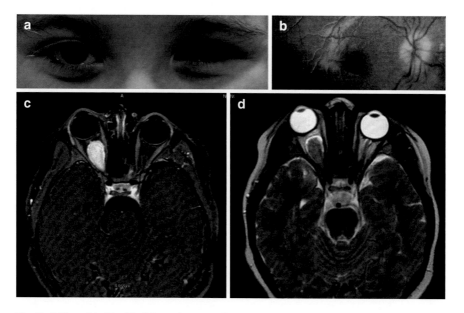

Fig. 2 6-Year-old girl with right optic nerve glioma presented with mild proptosis (**a**), decreased visual acuity, afferent pupillary defect, and disc edema (**b**). MRI shows fusiform right optic nerve lesion, which is showing contrast enhancement on T1 (**c**) and isointense on T2 sequence (**d**)

acuity loss during the following year. DTI allows identification and quantitation of white matter pathways, including optic nerves, tracts, and radiations [16].

As research continues to be conducted on the best imaging techniques, MRI continues to be the standard of care for imaging of OPGs when it is necessitated.

Recommendations for Management

Management options for OPGs include observation, chemotherapy, radiation, or surgery (Table 2). Choosing a treatment is often a difficult decision due to the unpredictable course of the tumor. Parsa et al. reported spontaneous regression in 12 out of the 13 eyes with improvement in visual function [17]. Smaller, asymptomatic tumors can be observed with periodic surveillance as per protocol. Considering that only one-third of OPGs progress, intervention is considered in patients when symptomatic. Indications for treatment include visual deterioration, tumor growth, increase in enhancement of MRI, visual field loss, endocrine dysfunction, hydrocephalus, or mass effect [18]. Liu et al. state that optic nerve gliomas without chiasmal involvement at presentation are more likely to remain localized without extension to the chiasm. Treatment for these patients for possible extension into chiasm is unwarranted.

Initiation of nonsurgical treatment is recommended in the case of clear evidence of bilateral visual deterioration. This can take the form of chemotherapy or radiation. A child with low vision unilaterally at presentation can still be observed if assessment in the child is reliable and they can be followed up closely every 1–2 months until further progressive deterioration is documented.

Chemotherapy is considered the primary treatment option in progressive OPG (documented as clinical or radiologic deterioration from baseline) of the chiasma or posterior optic pathway, when associated with NF1. In patients without NF1, a biopsy should be considered to ascertain the diagnosis. If a diagnosis of pilocytic astrocytoma is made, then chemotherapy is the option in symptomatic patients. A

Table 2 Treatment strategies for optic pathway gliomas

Chemotherapy
• Carboplatin and vincristine
• Vinblastine
• Cisplatin
• Cyclophosphamide
• Bevacizumab
• Temozolomide
• Cisplatin-etoposide-ifosfamide
• 6-Thioguanine-procarbazine-vincristine-lomustine
Radiation
• Fractioned stereotactic radiotherapy
• Stereotactic brachytherapy
• External fractioned radiotherapy
• Re-radiation

tumor with any other pathologic diagnosis in the optic pathway should be managed in a similar fashion to tumors of the same etiology arising elsewhere in CNS with chemotherapy or radiation [19].

The non-NF1 tumors involving the chiasm or hypothalamus are known to be chronically relapsing tumors which can eventually enter a static phase. Hence the general consensus in treatment of these tumors is to wait till tumor progression [20].

Studies have demonstrated that the risk of vision loss is higher in more posteriorly located tumors and in older individuals and hence it is recommended that children with posteriorly located tumors have a close follow-up and visual assessment till the age of 18.

Surgery is considered in patients of glioma involving optic nerve when they present with proptosis, mass effect, or significant deterioration of vision [21]. In chiasm involving tumors, surgery is used as the primary mode of management only for exophytic chiasmatic tumors, large tumors for de-bulking, or hydrocephalus [22]. These patients require close follow-up with two monthly scans for at least 6 months.

A multicenter retrospective cohort study aimed at determining the natural history of optic nerve gliomas found that during a mean follow-up of 5.6 years, 59% of the tumors progressed, 23% remained stable, and 18% (all with neurofibromatosis type 1) displayed some degree of spontaneous regression [23]. The authors concluded that radiological progression and visual deterioration occur in greater percentages in NF1 than in the general population of patients with OPGs. Response to chemotherapy may be better in this group, and its use should be considered early in the course of the disease.

Based on the Warburg hypothesis, mouse studies have shown regression of gliomas in response to ketogenic diet [24]. This is based on the theory that tumor cells thrive mainly on glycolysis for nutrition.

Radiation

Radiation therapy has not been recommended for treatment of OPG for quite some time now due to the risk of developing secondary tumors especially in children younger than the age of 5. The optic pathway glioma taskforce consensus report states that various studies suggested that radiotherapy appeared to improve the 5- and 10-year disease-free rates in patients with progressive gliomas. At 20 years, however, the overall disease-free survival rates are essentially equivalent between the patients who were treated with radiotherapy and those who were not [25].

Radiation therapy continues to have a role in the treatment for OPGs when it is refractive to other treatments such as chemotherapy. Combs et al. described fractionated stereotactic radiotherapy (FSRT) which was well tolerated in children and could be considered in unresectable tumors involving the chiasm. The 5-year survival rate after FSRT was 90%, and there were no secondary malignancies during this period [26]. It is important to note the short follow-up period in this study. FSRT as opposed to conventional radiotherapy has the ability to deliver a high-dose radiation to the tumor while sparing the normal brain tissue.

Table 3 Prognostic score to predict the outcome following re-irradiation

Prognostic factor	Subgroups	Value for prognostic score
Histology	WHO Grade IV	2
	WHO Grade III	1
	WHO Grade II	0
Age	<50 years	0
	>50 years	1
Time between RT and re-RT	<12 months	1
	>12 months	0

Reproduced from Kerstin A. Kessel, Josefine Hesse, Christoph Straube. Validation of an established prognostic score after re-irradiation of recurrent glioma. Acta Oncologica. 2017;56(3) [29]

Muller et al. published a subgroup analysis from the low-grade glioma (LGG) trial in 1996 on patients who underwent either stereotactic brachytherapy (SBT) or external fractionated radiotherapy (EBRT). He reported a 10-year overall survival rate and progression-free survival (PFS) rate of 97% and 70%, respectively. There was no significant difference in either the SBT or the EBRT groups. The overall dose required was effectively reduced with these techniques without jeopardizing tumor control [27].

Coombs et al. also re-irradiated gliomas with signs of malignant transformation when the tumors were unifocal and contrast enhancing with a maximal diameter of 4 cm. He developed a prognostic score to predict the outcome following re-irradiation which consisted of scoring based on the histology of tumor, the age of patient, and the time since previous radiation. The additive score was then generated using the three factors on the scale (range 0–4 points). Patients that scored 3–4 represented the worst outcome, and patients that scored 0 had the best outcome after re-irradiation. For treatment decisions, patients scoring 0–2 present a clear benefit from re-irradiation over those who had a higher score [28]. It should be noted that the histology of grade IV tumors, i.e., glioblastomas, has a higher score and this itself has a poor prognosis as an independent factor. This scoring system was later validated by Kessel et al. in an independent large cohort of 199 patients who underwent re-irradiation (Table 3) [29].

Chemotherapy

Results from the multicenter treatment trial of LGG in 1996 showed that chemotherapy with carboplatin and vincristine in gliomas involving the chiasma or hypothalamus is an effective therapy to delay any need for radiotherapy with an overall survival of 93% and radiotherapy-free survival of 83%. However, the conventional use of these agents has been reported to have a poorer response in children less than 1 year of age. Patients less than 1 year old have to adapt their treatment with the addition of another drug or a change in the chemotherapy regimen to improve outcomes in that patient population [30–32].

Some centers have reported up to 30% of children with OPGs having tumor progression despite first-line management with the standard chemo regimen. Azizi et al. evaluated the next line of management for these patients using Web-based questionnaire to members of SIOPE (Societé Internationale d'Oncologie Pédiatrique) brain tumor group. Components suggested for second line were vinblastine (62%), cisplatin (34%), and cyclophosphamide (26%). Bevacizumab (BVZ) was considered a suitable drug as a third line of chemotherapy, often with irinotecan and vinblastine, and has had favorable outcome [33, 34]. In addition to systemic therapy 38% of respondents would consider a neurosurgical option (if safely feasible) in combination with further chemotherapy [33]. A majority of the respondents in this study also stated that they would not use radiotherapy as a second- or third-line option upon failure of chemotherapy. Radiotherapy was considered as an option only after failure of the second- or third-line chemo drugs, and only once the children were older than age 7 [33].

Reports from a RCT involving 18 institutions and 11 countries to investigate the addition of etoposide by the International Society of Pediatric Oncology-Low Grade Glioma (SIOP LGG) Committee concluded that addition of etoposide to the standard regimen of carboplatin and vincristine did not significantly alter the 5-year overall survival or disease-free progression [35].

Bavle et al. described the use of BRAF inhibitor (dabrafenib) in the treatment of a patient with disseminated OPG with a BRAFv600e mutation refractory to MEK inhibition (selumetinib) [36].

A multicenter retrospective analysis of visual outcomes in children with NF1-associated OPG following carboplatin-based chemotherapy regimens reported that one-third of children had visual acuity improvement and another 40% had stable acuity. They concluded that tumor location was the most important prognostic factor to predict visual outcomes [18]. Prior studies had focused on radiologic progression for response of chemotherapy, which is now considered a poor predictor for outcomes. Therapy and follow-up should focus on visual changes as an outcome measure.

Other agents that are being used for chemotherapy include temozolomide [37], cisplatin-etoposide-ifosfamide (PEI), and 6-thioguanine-procarbazine-vincristine-CCNU (TPVC) [30]. Chemotherapy, when used as second-line management, is known to be equally effective as the first line and is known to have a 5-year overall survival and progression-free survival of 86 ± 6% and 37 ± 8%, respectively [38]. These values are comparable to first-line chemotherapy. A randomized control trial comparing the chemotherapy regimens of vincristine with carboplatin (CV) to TPCV (thioguanine, procarbazine, lomustine, and vincristine) reported that the 5-year event-free survival (EFS) was 39% ± 4% for CV and 52% ± 5% for TPCV. EFS with the TPCV regimen was similar to that of CV in the first 2 years, but the EFS was higher in the long term for TPCV.

The main side effects of using chemotherapy include an allergic response, a drug hypersensitivity, myelosuppression, bleeding, a higher rate of infection, and other drug-specific side effects such as hemorrhagic cystitis with the use of cyclophosphamide and neuropathy with Vinca alkaloids (vincristine).

Role and Evolution of Surgery in OPG

Biopsy in an OPG is considered only in radiologically atypical tumors, usually only in NF-1-negative patients, and only if it can be done safely and avoid damage to any neighboring structures. Suitable methods of collecting the biopsy include endoscopic biopsy, stereotactic biopsy, and open biopsy via craniotomy [39].

Surgery as a treatment is used in OPG when they involve optic chiasma or hypothalamus for de-bulking the tumor when they are symptomatic. A VP shunt can also be planned in the case of hydrocephalus and is a relatively safe procedure [40]. Though a total tumor resection of low-grade gliomas is associated with better 5-year survival rate there is always a potential risk of damage to vital structures. Gooden et al. reported an overall survival of 92% in patients who underwent primary surgery for tumors involving the chiasma or hypothalamus, with or without adjuvant therapy [41]. A more recent paper based on a retrospective analysis of children who underwent surgery for symptomatic OPG by Liu et al. reported the 5-year overall survival rate (OS) and progression-free survival rate (PFS) of 84.1% and 70.6%, respectively. The majority of the patients had a partial resection of tumor with the primary intent of de-bulking and all the patients received chemotherapy after surgery. Also, children >5 years old received 3D conformal radiotherapy and this subset of patients were reported to have a better OS and PFS when compared to those who did not.

Recently the use of intraoperative imaging in the form of ultrasound, CT, or MRI has emerged as a very useful tool to guide surgeons to enhance the possibility of maximal tumor bulk resection while preserving the vital surrounding structures. Ulrich et al. reported a resection rate of 82% while using 3D real-time USG intraoperatively. This technique could be supplemented with the use of neurosurgical navigation systems. Ultrasound has limitations in the fact that it is highly operator dependent and intraoperative spatial orientation could be cumbersome. However, it could be significantly cost effective and is easily installed. Use of intraoperative CT is not recommended in pediatric population due to exposure to radiation [41].

Another useful tool that has emerged is the use of intraoperative MRI [42]. It reduces the rate of re-surgery by around 7–10% by allowing maximal resection at a single sitting. It helps to localize residual tumors in planned complete tumor resections and their proximity to surrounding vital tissue. This allows the surgeon to plan accordingly to achieve maximal benefit with minimal neurological compromise [43, 44]. Although great in theory, this leads to greater acquisition time as well as higher costs.

Genetics and Possible Future Pathways for Treatment

Genetic research is continuingly being done in search for treatments that can possibly target one specific factor or pathway that would allow patients to theoretically have a smaller array of side effects compared to using chemo- or radiation therapy. Rodriguez et al. investigated BRAF mutations and the MAPK pathway in optic gliomas as possible targets for new therapy of optic nerve gliomas [45]. OPGs have also been found to be associated with activation of the mTOR/Akt pathway and inhibition of this pathway as a possible therapeutic agent was investigated in phase 2 trials with the use of everolimus in chemotherapy-resistant radiographically progressive pediatric low-grade gliomas. This has shown promise with significant tumor stability during treatment [46]. Decreased tumor perfusion is also seen, which is a positive effect of these drugs that could be used as marker to document tumor response with angiography. Cabezas et al. found heterogeneity among the tumors with activation of either mTORC1 or mTORC2 pediatric low-grade gliomas, which could probably explain variability of response of these tumors when a single pathway is targeted [47]. Essentially, the mTOR is a protein kinase which can control cell growth and proliferation in response to nutrients and growth factors and is frequently dysregulated in cancers [48]. These studies are encouraging and suggest that mTOR inhibition may become an important component of pediatric low-grade glioma treatment.

Key Points
- Optic pathways are clinically seen in 1–5% of neurofibromatosis 1 patients and is radiologically evident in 15%.
- Ophthalmic surveillance is essential to rule out a progressive optic pathway glioma.
- MRI is the primary mode of diagnosis and serial MRI could be necessary till age 8 years to rule out progression.
- Treatment options include surgery, chemotherapy, and radiation with lot of future treatment options available involving the mTOR pathway.

Acknowledgment This work was supported in part by an unrestricted institutional grant from Research to Prevent Blindness, NY, NY.

References

1. Dutton JJ. Gliomas of the anterior visual pathway. Surv Ophthalmol. 1994;38(5):427–52.
2. Wilhelm H. Primary optic nerve tumours. Curr Opin Neurol. 2009;22:11–8.
3. Robert-Boire V, Rosca L, Samson Y, Ospina LH, Perreault S. Clinical presentation and outcome of patients with optic pathway glioma. Pediatr Neurol. 2017;75:55–60.
4. Toledano H, Muhsinoglu O, Luckman J, Goldenberg-Cohen N, Michowiz S. Acquired nystagmus as the initial presenting sign of chiasmal glioma in young children. Eur J Paediatr Neurol. 2015;19(6):694–700. https://doi.org/10.1016/j.ejpn.2015.06.007. Epub 2015 Jul 9.

5. Silverman B, Listernick R, Charrow J. Precocious puberty in children with neurofibromatosis type 1. J Pediatr. 1995;126:364–7.
6. Sani I, Albanese A. Endocrine long-term follow-up of children with neurofibromatosis type 1 and optic pathway glioma. Horm Res Paediatr. 2017;87(3):179–88. https://doi.org/10.1159/000458525. Epub 2017 Mar 27.
7. Parsa CF, Hoyt CS. Spontaneous regression of optic gliomas: thirteen cases documented by serial neuroimaging. Arch Ophthalmol. 2001;119(4):516–2.
8. Liu GT, Malloy P, Needle M, Phillips P. Optic gliomas in neurofibromatosis type 1: role of visual evoked potentials. Pediatr Neurol. 1995;12:89–90.
9. Listernick R, Ferner RE, Liu GT, Gutmann DH. Optic pathway gliomas in neurofibromatosis-1: controversies and recommendations. Ann Neurol. 2007;61:189–98.
10. Stokland T, et al. A multivariate analysis of factors determining tumor progression in childhood low-grade glioma: a population-based cohort study (CCLG CNS9702). Neuro-Oncology. 2010;12(12):1257–68. PMC. Web. 8 Jan. 2018.
11. Diggs KA. Sex is a major determinant of neuronal dysfunction in neurofibromatosis type 1. Ann Neurol. 2014;75(2):309–16. Wiley 2014-2 0364-5134.
12. Hersh JH, American Academy of Pediatrics Committee on Genetics. Health supervision for children with neurofibromatosis. Pediatrics. 2008;121:633–42. https://doi.org/10.1542/peds.2007-3364.
13. Segal L, Darvish-Zargar M, Dilenge ME, Ortenberg J, Polomeno RC. Optic pathway gliomas in patients with neurofibromatosis type 1: follow-up of 44 patients. J AAPOS. 2010;14:155–8.
14. Yeom KW, Lober RM, Andre JB. Prognostic role for diffusion-weighted imaging of pediatric optic pathway glioma. J Neuro-Oncol. 2013;113:479.
15. Purohit BS, et al. Orbital tumours and tumour-like lesions: exploring the armamentarium of multiparametric imaging. Insights Imaging. 2016;7(1):43–68.
16. Kennedy de Blank PM, Jeffrey Berman I, Liu G, Leslie Roberts TP, Fisher M. Fractional anisotropy of the optic radiations is associated with visual acuity loss in optic pathway gliomas of neurofibromatosis type 1. Neuro-Oncology. 2013;15(8):1088–95.
17. Parsa CF, Hoyt CS, Lesser RL, et al. Spontaneous regression of optic gliomas: thirteen cases documented by serial neuroimaging. Arch Ophthalmol. 2001;119:516–29.
18. Fisher M, Loguidice M, Gutmann D, Listernickr R, Liu G. Visual outcomes in children with neurofibromatosis type 1–associated optic pathway glioma following chemotherapy: a multicenter retrospective analysis. Neuro-Oncology. 2012;14(6):790–7.
19. Thomas RP, Gibbs IC, Xu LW. Treatment options for optic pathway gliomas. Curr Treat Options Neurol. 2015;17:2.
20. Stokland T, Liu JF, Ironside JW, Ellison DW, Taylor R, Robinson KJ, Picton SV, Walker DA. A multivariate analysis of factors determining tumor progression in childhood low-grade glioma: a population-based cohort study (CCLG CNS9702). Neuro-Oncology. 2010;12(12):1257–68.
21. Balcer LJ, Liu GT, Heller G, et al. Visual loss in children with neurofibromatosis type 1 and optic pathway gliomas: relation to tumor location by magnetic resonance imaging. Am J Ophthalmol. 2001;131:442–5.
22. Astrup J. Natural history and clinical management of optic pathway glioma. Br J Neurosurg. 2003;17:327–35.
23. Shofty B, Ben-Sira K, Jallo G, Isolated Optic Nerve Abnormalities (IONA) Collaboration. Isolated optic nerve gliomas: a multicenter historical cohort study. J Neurosurg Pediatr. 2017;20(6):549–55.
24. Stafford P, Abdelwahab MG, do Kim Y, Preul MC, Rho JM, Scheck AC. The ketogenic diet reverses gene expression patterns and reduces reactive oxygen species levels when used as an adjuvant therapy for glioma. Nutr Metab (Lond). 2010;10(7):74.
25. Listernick R. Optic pathway gliomas in children with neurofibromatosis 1: consensus statement from the NF1 Optic Pathway Glioma Task Force. Ann Neurol. 1997;41(2):143–9. Wiley 1997-2;0364-5134.
26. Combs SE, Schulz-Ertner D, Moschos D, Thilmann C, Huber PE, Debus J. Fractionated stereotactic radiotherapy of optic pathway gliomas: tolerance and long-term outcome. Int J Radiat Oncol Biol Phys. 2005;62:814–9.

27. Müller K. Radiotherapy in pediatric pilocytic astrocytomas. A subgroup analysis within the prospective multicenter study HIT-LGG 1996 by the German Society of Pediatric Oncology and Hematology (GPOH). Strahlenther Onkol. 2013;189(8):647–55. Springer 2013-8;0179-7158.
28. Combs SE, Edler L, Rausch R, Welzel T, Wick W, Debus J. Generation and validation of a prognostic score to predict outcome after re-irradiation of recurrent glioma. Acta Oncol. 2013;52(1):147–52.
29. Kessel KA, Hesse J, Straube C. Validation of an established prognostic score after re-irradiation of recurrent glioma. Acta Oncol. 2017;56(3):422–6.
30. Mirow C, Pietsch T, Berkefeld S, Kwiecien R, Warmuth-Metz M, Falkenstein. Children <1 year show an inferior outcome when treated according to the traditional LGG treatment strategy: a report from the German multicenter trial HIT-LGG 1996 for children with low grade glioma (LGG). Pediatr Blood Cancer. 2014;61:457–63.
31. Ater J, Zhou T, Homes E, et al. Randomized study of two chemotherapy regimens for treatment of low-grade glioma in young children: a report from the Children's Oncology Group. J Clin Oncol. 2012;30:2641–7.
32. Ater JL, Holmes E, Zhoy T, et al. Randomized study of two chemotherapy regimens for low grade glioma in young children: results of COG protocol A9952. Pediatr Blood Cancer. 2008;53.
33. Azizi AA, Schouten-van Meeteren AYN. Current and emerging treatment strategies for children with progressive chiasmatic-hypothalamic glioma diagnosed as infants: a web-based survey. J Neuro-Oncol. 2018;136:127.
34. Packer RJ, Jakacki R, Horn M, Rood B, Vezina G, MacDonald T, Fisher MJ, Cohen B. Objective response of multiply recurrent low-grade gliomas to bevacizumab and irinotecan. Pediatr Blood Cancer. 2009;52(7):791–5.
35. Gnekow AK, Walker DA, Kandels D, Picton S. A European randomised controlled trial of the addition of etoposide to standard vincristine and carboplatin induction as part of an 18-month treatment programme for childhood (≤16 years) low grade glioma—a final report. Eur J Cancer. 2017;81:206–25.
36. Bavle A, Jones J, Lin FY, Malphrus A, Adesina A, Su J. Dramatic clinical and radiographic response to BRAF inhibition in a patient with progressive disseminated optic pathway glioma refractory to MEK inhibition. Pediatr Hematol Oncol. 2017;34(4):254–9.
37. Gururangan S, Fisher MJ, Allen JC, Herndon JE II, Quinn JA, Reardon DA, et al. Temozolomide in children with progressive low-grade glioma. Neuro-Oncology. 2007;9(2):161–8.
38. Scheinemann K, Bartels U, Tsangaris E, Hawkins C, Huang A, Dirks P, Fried I, Bouffet E, Tabori U. Feasibility and efficacy of repeated chemotherapy for progressive pediatric low-grade gliomas. Pediatr Blood Cancer. 2011;57:84–8.
39. Walker DA, Liu J, Kieran M, Jabado N, Picton S, Packer R, et al. A multi-disciplinary consensus statement concerning surgical approaches to low-grade, high-grade astrocytomas and diffuse intrinsic pontine gliomas in childhood (CPN Paris 2011) using the Delphi method. Neuro-Oncology. 2013;15:462–8.
40. Liu Y, et al. Analysis of survival prognosis for children with symptomatic optic pathway gliomas who received surgery. World Neurosurg. 2018;109:e1–e15. https://doi.org/10.1016/j.wneu.2017.09.144.
41. Ulrich NH, Burkhardt JK, Serra C, et al. Resection of pediatric intracerebral tumors with the aid of intraoperative real-time 3-D ultrasound. Childs Nerv Syst. 2012;28:101–9.
42. Goodden J, Pizer B, Pettorini B, Williams D, Blair J, Didi M, Thorp N, Mallucci C. The role of surgery in optic pathway/hypothalamic gliomas in children. J Neurosurg Pediatr. 2014;13(1):1–12.
43. Shah MN, Leonard JR, Inder G. Intraoperative magnetic resonance imaging to reduce the rate of early reoperation for lesion resection in pediatric neurosurgery. J Neurosurg Pediatr. 2012;9:259–64.
44. Giordano M, Arraez C, Samii A, et al. Childs Nerv Syst. 2016;32:1915.
45. Rodriguez FJ, Ligon AH, Horkayne-Szakaly I, et al. *BRAF* duplications and MAPK pathway activation are frequent in gliomas of the optic nerve proper. J Neuropathol Exp Neurol. 2012;71(9):789–94.

46. Segal D, Gardner S, Allen J, Karajannis M. EPT-21 Efficacy of everolimus in pediatric brain tumors: a single-institution patient series. Neuro-Oncology. 2016;18(Suppl 3):iii28.
47. Hütt-Cabezas M, et al. Activation of mTORC1/mTORC2 signaling in pediatric low-grade glioma and pilocytic astrocytoma reveals mTOR as a therapeutic target. Neuro-Oncology. 2013;15(12):1604–14.
48. Asati V, Mahapatra DK, Bharti SK. PI3K/Akt/mTOR and Ras/Raf/MEK/ERK signaling pathways inhibitors as anticancer agents: structural and pharmacological perspectives. Eur J Med Chem. 2016;109:314–41.

Current Management of Ocular Surface Squamous Neoplasia (OSSN)

S. Madison Duff, Niloofar Piri, and Hossein Asghari

Introduction

Ocular surface squamous neoplasia (OSSN), a term originating from [1] paper, describes a spectrum of "ocular surface" premalignant and malignant lesions (dysplastic, carcinoma in situ, and invasive carcinoma) of squamous cell etiology.

It is the most common nonpigmented tumor of the conjunctiva.

- For the purpose of this chapter, treatment of preinvasive CIN and invasive squamous carcinoma will be discussed.
  - **Preinvasive lesions**: Conjunctival/corneal intraepithelial neoplasms (CIN I, CIN II, CIN III) (Fig. 1b):
    - o CIN I: Dysplasia of the lower 1/3 of the conjunctiva
    - o CIN II: Dysplasia extending to the middle third
    - o CIN III: Full-thickness dysplasia [in situ]
  - **Malignant or invasive lesions**: Squamous carcinoma (Fig. 1a) and mucoepidermoid carcinoma
- OSSN typically originates in the conjunctiva and extends across the limbus to invade the cornea, but may rarely originate in the cornea [2]. This neoplasia primarily spreads by local invasion. Intraocular invasion and metastasis are uncommon, but may occur with delays in medical treatment [3].
- Historically, wide surgical excision with or without supplemental cryotherapy was a paragon of therapy, but it has changed significantly in the past two decades due to improved diagnostic capabilities and a shift towards medical management of these tumors.

S. M. Duff · N. Piri · H. Asghari (✉)
University of Louisville Ophthalmology, Louisville, KY, USA
e-mail: smduff05@cardmail.louisville.edu; niloofar.piri@louisville.edu; h0asgh01@exchange.louisville.edu

© Springer Nature Singapore Pte Ltd. 2019
A. Ramasubramanian (ed.), *Ocular Oncology*, Current Practices in Ophthalmology, https://doi.org/10.1007/978-981-13-7538-5_5

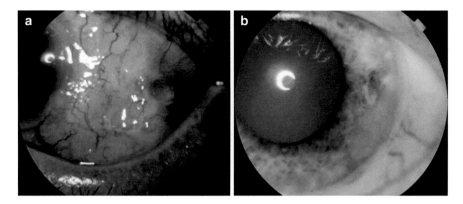

Fig. 1 (a) Squamous cell carcinoma with scleral invasion. (b) Conjunctival intraepithelial neoplasia (image courtesy—Aparna Ramasubramanian, MD)

- The **OPTIMAL TREATMENT PLAN** is individualized, depending on the size and locations of the tumor, depth of invasion, and prior treatment attempts, in addition to the individual patient's comfort level and willingness to comply.

Medical Therapy of OSSN

- Medical treatment of OSSN consists primarily of topical IFN-α2b, mitomycin (MMC), and 5-fluorouracil (5-FU) that have shown themselves to be clinically effective

◊ If tumor's largest diameter
    < 3 clock hours   → Excisional biopsy
◊ If tumor's largest diameter
    3 to 6 clock hours   → 1] Excisional biopsy [to confirm diagnosis + determine invasiveness]
    • Pre-invasive   → 2] Topical Medical Therapy
    • Invasive   → 2] Consider Trial of Topical or Injected Medical Therapy for complete resolution or chemo-reduction
       ° If tumor remains   → 3] Wide "No Touch" Excision + Cryotherapy Surrounding Excision

         ° If corneal component   → Alcohol Epitheliectomy (Palmar, 2014)
         ° If invading scleral component → Sclerectomy with Adjunctive Alcohol Application to Base (Tananuvat, 2012)
         ° Depending on size of conjunctival defect → Tissue Replacement

◊ If tumor's largest diameter
    > 6 clock hours   → 1] Trial of Topical or Injected Medical Therapy for chemo-reduction (or possible complete eradiation)

    • For large invasive lesions
    that fail to respond   → 2] ° Palliative Treatment of Enucleation or Exenteration
                   ° Plaque Radiotherapy may be an alternative (Arepalli, 2014)

.

- Clinical Use
  - *Primary therapy*
    - o Certain agents may be effective in inducing tumor regression when used as a sole treatment for OSSN.
    - o Exclusive topical therapy is generally not recommended for invasive squamous cell carcinoma.
  - *Preoperative /neoadjuvant therapy*
    - o Topical agents may decrease a tumor's size prior to surgical treatment.
    - o Neoadjuvant therapy can be especially useful for diffuse OSSN.
  - *Intraoperative therapy*
    - o Topical therapy can be used intraoperatively as a substitute for cryotherapy.
  - *Postoperative therapy*
    - o Topical therapy may be used to reduce the risk of tumor recurrence, especially in cases of positive surgical margins, rather than necessitating a repeat surgical intervention.
- Relative indications for topical therapy in the treatment of noninvasive OSSN suggested by Sepulveda et al. [4]
  - >2 Quadrants of conjunctival involvement
  - >180° of limbal involvement
  - Extension into the clear cornea involving pupillary axis
  - Positive margins after excision
  - Patient unable to undergo surgery
- Advantages of Topical Medical Therapy
  - Treats the entire ocular surface, eliminating the necessity of ensuring clear surgical margins in a disease of microscopic dysplasia and varying borders
  - Reduces cost to the patient by avoiding surgical intervention primarily or with recurrence
- Disadvantages of Topical Medical Therapy
  - Compliance issues with regard to regimens frequently requiring multiple eye drops each day
  - Long-term consequences of the agents on the surface of the eye remain largely unknown
  - Regimens for each agent are still being cultivated
  - May fail to completely eradicate the tumor
  - Clinical toxicities and complications exist that are specific to each agent

Mitomycin C (MMC)

- An alkylating agent isolated from Streptomyces species that was first reported efficacious for ocular surface squamous neoplasia in 1994 by Frucht-Perry and Rozenman [5]

Mechanism of Action
- Produces DNA cross-linking by alkylation, inhibiting DNA synthesis to target rapidly growing cells, especially in the intracellular hypoxic environments of tumor cells [2]
- Acts primarily in an aerobic environment when used topically to generate free radicals that result in lipid peroxidation, thus becoming cytotoxic to the neoplasia [6]

Application and Dosing
- MMC has been proven efficacious when used exclusively [5], preoperatively as chemoreduction [7], and following surgical excision to reduce the rate of recurrence in conjunctival-corneal intraepithelial neoplasia [8].
- MMC preserves its activity for longer when refrigerated at 4 °C [4], but may require weekly replacement [9].
- MMC is used at 0.02 or 0.04% concentrations.
- As there remain no studies directly comparing different concentrations of MMC on altered schedules, different protocols are being used. The lower concentration [0.02%] may be used q.i.d. for 2 weeks, followed by a period of rest prior to repetition [10] or continuously till regression [11]. The higher concentration [0.04%] is typically administered q.i.d. for 1 week, followed by 3 weeks off treatment [9], but may be administered for longer [12].
- As a general rule, breaks in treatment are thought to reduce side effects [13] and higher concentrations tend to be used for shorter interval than lower concentrations for the same reason.

Noteworthy Published Studies
- *Wilson and colleagues* in 1997 showed clinical regression of six of seven eyes with CIN when using 0.04% topical mitomycin [14]
- *Rozenman and Frucht-Pery* in 2000 showed both 0.02 and 0.04% concentrations of MMC to be effective in small (<8 mm in diameter) CIN treatment, but demonstrated that repeated cycles may be required [10].
- *Frucht-Pery et al.'s* 2002 paper presented five patients that had histologically proven, incompletely excised conjunctival SCC that were postoperatively managed with three cycles of 14-day treatments of MMC. After repeat excision of the surrounding conjunctiva, all biopsies were negative for malignant cells [15].
- *Shields, Naseripour, and Shields* reported in 2002 ten patients with conjunctival and corneal SCC that were treated with topical mitomycin C as a primary treatment. Each patient had complete tumor response and regression, with no recurrences in the mean follow-up time of 22 months [16].
- *Chen and colleagues* reported in 2004 27 ocular surface squamous cell neoplasias that were treated with surgical excision. Only 17 of the neoplasias were treated with adjuvant cryotherapy, but all of the neoplasias were treated with two or three 1-week therapy cycles of MMC. At a mean follow-up of 27 months, zero recurrences occurred [17].

- *Prabhasawat and colleagues* treated seven patients and found that the lower concentration of 0.02% MMC was effective in treating both CIN and SCC in six of the seven patients as a primary treatment [11].
- *Shields and colleagues* suggested in a 2005 paper that topical mitomycin C be used as a neoadjuvant chemotherapeutic agent prior to thickened (>4 mm) or extensive conjunctival SCC surgical treatment to allow for a less extensive resection [7].
- *Gupta and Muecke*'s 2010 paper found no recurrence in 73 eyes of noninvasive OSSN when surgical excision and cryotherapy were followed by topical MMC, thus recommending MCC's use as adjuvant therapy. Additionally, diffuse disease was stated to benefit from sole MMC therapy; however, close follow-up was recommended due to persistent or recurrent neoplasia [8].
- *Birkholz and colleagues'* retrospective 2011 case review suggested that even if surgical margins were histopathologically negative, adjunctive (intraoperative or postoperative) use of mitomycin C was beneficial in significantly reducing the prevalence of recurrence [18].

Side Effects
- Toxicity of the ocular surface occurring from MMC appears to occur in a dosage-dependent pattern [11].
- Drug-related complications may occur in as high as >50% of patients being treated with MMC, but serious long-term complications are rare [19].
- Common side effects:
  - Conjunctival hyperemia
  - Allergic reactions (lid swelling)
  - Allergic conjunctivitis
  - Punctal stenosis
  - Toxic epitheliopathy [9]
- Long-term side effects:
  - Recurrent corneal erosion
  - Limbal stem cell deficiency [20]
- Cellular changes from mitomycin C have been shown to persist at least 8 months following therapy and have been stated to mimic the effects of ionizing radiation [21].
- Due to the possibility of ocular surface toxicity, MMC is contraindicated in cases of dry eye or atopy [4].
- To avoid the risk of corneo-scleral melting, topical therapy should be postponed post-biopsy to allow for complete healing [4].
- It is recommended to place punctal plugs in both upper and lower puncti to prevent punctal stenosis [4]. However, some argue that exposure of lacrimal system to MMC is important in reducing the likelihood of tumor recurrence in this place (Russell 2010).

Efficacy
- MMC has been shown to be very effective, especially in localized lesions (0 recurrence in localized lesions, 30% recurrence in diffuse lesions) [8].
- Although efficacy rates fluctuate based on sample sizes, differing concentrations, and treatment schedules, MMC has an overall efficacy in resolution rates of between 82 and 100% [20].
- Major limitation of topical MMC is pain and toxic epitheliopathy.

5-Fluorouracil (5-FU)

- 5-FU is a pyrimidine analog that was first utilized for OSSN by de Keizer and colleagues in 1986 [22].

Mechanism of Action
- This antimetabolite acts against the enzyme thymidylate synthetase, thus inhibiting the production and incorporation of thymidine into DNA, inhibiting RNA synthesis, and causing cell death.

Application and Dosing
- The most commonly used protocol is administration of 1% 5-FU topically four times a day for 4–7 days, followed by 1 month off [23].

Noteworthy Published Studies
- *De Keizer and colleagues* showed 5-FU to be an effective treatment in two patients with noninvasive OSSN [22].
- *Yeatts and colleagues* utilized 1% 5-FU topically q.i.d. for 2–3 weeks in six patients with OSSN. One patient ultimately required exenteration and one required surgical excision, but four remained tumor free for a range of 10–30 months [24].
- In 2000, *Yeatts and colleagues* attempted topical treatment with 1% 5-FU given q.i.d. for 2–4 days, and repeated at 30–45-day intervals, in seven patients. Four patients had no recurrence and the authors concluded that pulsed dosing may be both effective and well tolerated [23].
- *Midena and colleagues* presented eight cases of OSSN treated with 1% topical 5-FU q.i.d. for 4 weeks. In a mean follow-up of 27 months, only one patient required a repeat course of 5-FU [25].
- *Rudkin and Muecke* in 2011 reported 65 cases of OSSN that were treated with excision, cryotherapy, and adjuvant 5-FU 1% q.i.d. for 2 weeks. One case (1.5%) had recurrence in 12 months and four patients stopped the 5-FU 1% prematurely due to local side effects [26].
- *Parrozzani and colleagues* in 2017 showed 1% 5-FU q.i.d. for 4 weeks in 41 eyes to be effective for preinvasive OSSN, in addition to some invasive OSSN [27].

Side Effects
- Similar to MMC, but with less serious side effects:
  - Conjunctival hyperemia
  - Punctate epithelial erosions
  - Eyelid erythema and mild edema
- No long-term complications appeared with topical treatment [28].

Efficacy
- In studies of 44 patients and 41 patients treated with 1% 5-FU q.i.d., complete tumor regression was seen with 82% and 83% of OSSN, respectively [27, 29].

Interferon-α_{2b}

- A glycoprotein that was first utilized for ocular surface squamous neoplasia in 1994 by Maskin [30]

Mechanism of Action
- Although not fully understood, interferon-α2b modulates the immune system, is specifically thought to suppress IL-10 expression, and stimulates expression of IL-2 and IFNγ mRNA by tumor cells, making them prone to local immune system, thereby limiting their growth and invasion [4, 31].

Application and Dosing
- IFN-α2b may be given topically or as an injection (subconjunctival, perilesional, or intralesional).
- Topically the recommended dose is off-label use of one million IU/mL q.i.d. for 3–4 months. It needs compounding and refrigeration.
- As a subconjunctival injection, the dose is typically three million IU/mL, either three times a week or once a week, until tumor resolution. The preferred intervals for dosing remain undetermined [32].
- Intralesional IFN does not need to be compounded.

Noteworthy Published Studies
- *Maskin* treated a 55-year-old with epithelial dysplasia of the ocular surface who had already attempted excision with cryotherapy with topical recombinant interferon-alpha-2b treatment (one million U/mL b.i.d.) to complete resolution within 2 months [30].
- *Vann and Karp* reported in 1999 the combined use of subconjunctival/perilesional injection of recombinant IFN-α2b and subsequent topical IFN-α2b drops in six patients with histologically proven CIN. All patients showed complete resolution in 6 weeks and no recurrence in time of follow-up, 2–11 months [33].
- *Karp, Moore, and Rosa* published five case studies of patients with CIN in 2001 treated solely with topical IFN-α2b four times a day. One patient had a

recurrence at 1 year that was effectively treated with repeated topical IFN-α2b therapy [34].
- *Boehm and Huang* in 2004 described seven patients with CIN treated exclusively with topical IFN-α2b four times a day. Two patients had recurrences [35].
- *Galor and colleagues* in 2010 showed there to be no significant differences in the treatment of CIN with topical IFN-α2b at the typically used one million IU/mL dose and a three million IU/mL dose. This study also showed topical IFN-α2b to be an ineffective treatment for two cases of SCC [36].
- *Besley* et al. in 2014 showed topical IFN-α2b to be an effective treatment for OSSN after MMC therapy had failed to resolve the tumor [9].

Side Effects
- Topical IFN-α2b has been shown to be well tolerated, albeit it is expensive and requires both special compounding and subsequent refrigeration.
- Common side effects of topical therapy:
  - Mild irritation [32]
  - Follicular conjunctivitis [34]
- The main side effect of intralesional injection is influenza-like syndrome with fever and generalized malaise, which can be easily managed with acetaminophen after the injection and every 4-h PRN [32].

Efficacy
- *Schechter and colleagues* followed 28 eyes with OSSN treated solely with topical IFN-α2b. One eye did not have a full response (96.4% showed complete response). The remaining 27 eyes were followed for a range of 12–89 months. One eye (3.7%) had a recurrence during the follow-up [37].
- *Nanji* et al. reported in 2013 that across reviewed studies using topical IFN-α2b, the recurrence rate was 6% [38].
- Topical IFN-a2b appears to have a longer time for tumor resolution and remains more expensive than MMC and 5-FU, yet it may be better tolerated with less side effects [20].

Although IFN-a2b is more expensive, it is better tolerated with less side effects and is considered first-line therapy in cases that need topical treatment.

- *MMC is contraindicated in severe dry eye and atopy.*
- *When a patient is intolerant to one topical agent, different agents can be used.*
- *The best alternative is IFN-a2b given low-profile side effect.*

As none of these drugs are approved by FDA for treatment of OSSN, their use is considered off-label, and thus informed consent should be obtained from the patient.

Anti-vascular Endothelial Growth Factor

- Anti-VEGF is a humanized antibody against VEGF, a growth factor that is essential for vascular endothelial cell growth that results in angiogenesis.
- Utilization of anti-VEGF therapy in the treatment of OSSN remains limited.

Mechanism of Action
- Anti-VEGF agents inhibit neovascularization, which may explain why only vascular regions of the conjunctiva and not avascular corneal areas appear to respond to anti-VEGF therapy [39].

Application and Dosing
- Two agents, bevacizumab and ranibizumab, have been utilized for OSSN: bevacizumab has been used topically and as a subconjunctival injection, while ranibizumab solely as injection.
- Further exploration is required to determine the required dose and frequency of treatment.

Noteworthy Published Studies
- *Paul and Stone* used an intralesional injection of bevacizumab in a case of severe OSSN that had already failed other topical and intralesional chemotherapies. Bevacizumab failed to show any effect [40].
- Faramarzi and Feizi showed subconjunctival injections of bevacizumab to be beneficial in reducing OSSN size, but to be uneffective in the treatment of OSSN with corneal extension [39].
- *Özcan and colleagues* treated ten cases of OSSN with topical bevacizumab and concluded that topical bevacizumab may be utilized as an adjunctive therapy, but should not be utilized as the sole treatment of OSSN [20].
- *Asena and Dursun Altınors* used for the first time topical bevacizumab q.i.d. for 8 weeks in six eyes with OSSN. While two eyes did experience tumor resolution, four eyes experienced tumor reduction, but required surgical excision [41].
- *Finger and Chin* utilized subconjunctival ranibizumab in the treatment of SCC of the conjunctiva and cornea and found three of the patients to have a complete response [42].

Side Effects
- No significant local or systemic symptoms were observed with topical therapy [20] or subconjunctival injection [39].

Further comparative studies are needed to reveal safety and efficacy of topical anti-VEGF in the treatment of OSSN.

Surgical Treatment for OSSN

- Although topical therapies have become more popular in the last two decades, surgical excision remains the most important treatment option in the management of OSSN.
- A "no-touch" surgical excision with wide margins, followed by intraoperative double-freeze-thaw cryotherapy at the conjunctival margin and involved limbus and intraoperative alcohol epitheliectomy for the corneal component, remains the standard treatment.

If the excision is large, generally greater than 4 clock hours, tissue replacement becomes necessary [3] or prior topical therapy should be considered [43]. If the tumor is adherent, sclerectomy with adjunctive alcohol application to base is essential. Further local invasion may require enucleation or exenteration, although recent studies suggest that plaque radiotherapy may be attempted [44]. A sentinel node biopsy may become necessary to determine if neoplastic spread has already occurred.

"No-Touch" Technique [45]
- This technique, first described by Shields in the 1994 Lynn B. McMahan Lecture to describe the removal of conjunctival tumors, focuses on minimal manipulation of the tumor to prevent neoplastic cell seeding of adjacent tissue.
- In contrast to using forceps to elevate the lesion and removing the lesion with scissors, the excision should be attempted without touching the tumor with any instruments and the eye should be left dry until the tumor is completed excised [3].
- Retrobulbar anesthesia is preferred, as subconjunctival injection might blur the architecture of the tumor of emphasis.
- Excisional biopsy is preferred over an incisional biopsy.
- Bowman's layer may act as a natural barrier to invasion, and thus it is preserved.
- For a limbal tumor, treatment includes an alcohol epitheliectomy localized to the affected cornea, resection of the tumor with wide margins, and cryotherapy on the surrounding tissue margins.
- A wide surgical margin is defined as 4–5 mm in the case of conjunctival tumors [45]. This protects from recurrence, as seemingly uninvolved conjunctiva may contain neoplastic cells.
- Even with utilization of the "no-touch" technique, intraoperative cryotherapy, and intraoperative alcohol epitheliectomy, recurrence rates range from 15 to 52% [1].

Alcohol Corneal Epitheliectomy [45]
- A cotton-tipped applicator is soaked with absolute alcohol and applied to the corneal epithelium affected by the tumor. A suggested 2 mm of visibly normal corneal epithelium also receives the treatment.

Cryotherapy
- Intraoperatively, the cryoprobe and forceps are utilized to lift the conjunctival edge away from the sclera. The conjunctiva is frozen for 10–15 s, before thawing and being refrozen (double freeze-thaw). The cryoprobe is then advanced 3 mm along the conjunctival edge before repeating the double-freeze-thaw technique until the entire bulbar conjunctiva that previously surrounded the tumor has been treated [45].
- *Sudesh and colleagues* showed that the rate of recurrence decreased dramatically with the addition of intraoperative cryotherapy. In primary tumors, 28.5% of excised tumors, compared to 7.7% of tumors excised and treated with cryotherapy, exhibited recurrence. Differing recurrence rates were even more drastic in recurrent tumors [46].

Large Conjunctival Defects
- Defects too large to close primarily require a flap or graft. Options include a transpositional conjunctival flap, a mucous membrane autograft harvested from the opposite eye, a buccal mucosa graft, or an amniotic membrane transplant [3].
- In lesions larger than 10 mm, an amniotic membrane transplant may be preferred for conjunctival closure [47].

Invasion
- While OSSN typically remains superficial, 3–9% of cases may have intraocular invasion and 1–6% of cases may have orbital invasion [44].
- If OSSN invades deeply into the cornea, deep lamellar keratoplasty and scleroplasty are the surgical treatments of choice [1].
- Although plaque radiotherapy may be a new treatment option, intraocular or orbital invasion is frequently treated with enucleation or orbital exenteration [48].

Recurrence
- Negative surgical margins are key in preventing recurrence [21].
- In 1978, *Pizzarello and colleagues* noted that there was a 69% recurrence rate if neoplastic cells were left at the surgical margins [49].
- *Erie and colleagues* in 1986 noted that fully excised lesions with negative margins had a 5% recurrence rate, while incompletely excised lesions had a 53% recurrence rate [50].
- *Li and colleagues* in 2015 commented on the trend of physicians treating OSSN with topical therapy without a definitive diagnosis. They found that with excision and cryotherapy, recurrence rates, even with pathological evidence of tumor at the margins, were 7.1% at 1, 2, and 5 years, pointing out that the gold standard

of excision and cryotherapy provides good recurrence rates and a definitive diagnosis [51].

- In 2016, *Siedlecki and colleagues* used a literature-based decision analysis and concluded that surgical excision and IFN-a2b for surgical margins is the preferred strategy to minimize recurrence of OSSN [52].
- *Besley and colleagues* suggested that the majority of recurrences of OSSN (73%) occur within 2 years, and thus follow-ups should be more frequent in the first 2 years following treatment cessation [9].
- *Tabin and colleagues* in 1997 noted that recurrences have been seen as late as 11 years after surgical excision. Even with negative surgical margins, up to one-third of patients experience recurrence, and thus patients may require yearly follow-ups indefinitely [53].

- *If margins are positive after surgery, preferred treatment method is topical IFN-a2b for 1 month.*
- *The most common recurrence period is 2 years after surgery, during the time which more close monitoring is recommended.*

Radiation Treatment for OSSN

- Radiation therapy for OSSN has been used in the past, but due to the availability of alternative treatments and unwanted side effect it is not commonly used at this time in the treatment of OSSN.

Side Effects [1]
- Dry eye
- Cataracts
- Persistent scleral ulceration
- Symblepharon
- Corneal rupture [54]

Beta Radiation
- In 1976, Lommatzsch utilized beta-ray ocular applicators using strontium-90 and yttrium-90 to treat ten ocular SCCs and four CIN III tumors. Recurrence occurred in one patient who might have been inadequately treated [55].
- Kearsley and colleagues used surgical excision followed by beta radiation to treat "superficial conjunctival squamous cell cancer" [56].

Plaque Radiotherapy
- If OSSN becomes invasive, historically the treatment has been enucleation. *Arepalli and colleagues* treated 15 patients with invasive conjunctival SCC with plaque radiotherapy. Ten of the patients ultimately were able to avoid enucleation [44].

Photodynamic Therapy (PDT) for OSSN

- Initial results in the treatment of conjunctival OSSN were promising, but more investigation is necessary (Barebazetto 2004).

Application
- A photosensitizer is first administered. Verteporfin is typically utilized. This is followed by a light source, such as a light-emitting diode (LED) that emits red light in the case of verteporfin, to activate the porphyrin derivative at its specific wavelength.

Noteworthy Published Studies
- *Barbazetto and colleagues* utilized PDT in three patients with conjunctival OSSN and showed tumor regression in the irradiate areas of all three patients.
- *Ramasubramanian and colleagues* utilized PDT after corneal grafting and subsequent OSSN in a patient with preexisting corneal thinning that had already failed topical IFN-α2b. The patient showed complete tumor resolution with no recurrence in 8 months with PDT therapy [13].

Side Effects
- Minor headache [57]
- Local irritation [58]
- Conjunctival injection [58]
- Back pain (Barbazetto [58]

References

1. Lee GA, Hirst LW. Ocular surface squamous neoplasia. Surv Ophthalmol. 1995;39:429–50.
2. Basti S, Macsai MS. Ocular surface squamous neoplasia: a review. Cornea. 2003;22:687–704.
3. Tananuvat N, Lertprasertsuke N. Ocular surface squamous neoplasia. In: Srivastava S. Intraepithelial neoplasia; 2012. ISBN: 978–953–307-987-5. InTech. http://www.intechopen.com/books/intraepithelial-neoplasia/ocular-surface-squamous-neoplasia. Accessed 20 Jul 2017.
4. Sepulveda R, Pe'er J, Midena E, et al. Topical chemotherapy for ocular surface squamous neoplasia: current status. Br J Ophthalmol. 2010;94:532–5.
5. Frucht-Pery J, Rozenman Y. Mitomycin C therapy for corneal intraepithelial neoplasia. Am J Ophthalmol. 1994;117(2):164–8.
6. Verweij J, Pinedo HM. Mitomycin C: mechanism of action, usefulness and limitations. Anti-Cancer Drugs. 1990;1:5e13.
7. Shields CL, Demirci H, Marr BP, et al. Chemoreduction with topical mitomycin C prior to resection of extensive squamous cell carcinoma of the conjunctiva. Arch Ophthalmol. 2005;123:109–13.
8. Gupta A, Muecke J. Treatment of ocular surface squamous neoplasia with mitomycin C. Br J Ophthalmol. 2010;94:555–8.
9. Besley J, Pappalardo J, Lee GA, et al. Risk factors for ocular surface squamous neoplasia recurrence after treatment with topical mitomycin C and interferon alpha-2b. Am J Ophthalmol. 2014;157(2):287–93.
10. Rozenman Y, Frucht-Pery J. Treatment of conjunctival intraepithelial neoplasia with topical drops of mitomycin C. Cornea. 2000;19:1–6.

11. Prabhasawat P, Tarinvorakup P, Tesavibul N, et al. Topical 0.002% mitomycin C for the treatment of conjunctival-corneal intraepithelial neoplasia and squamous cell carcinoma. Cornea. 2005;24:443–8.

12. Russell HC, Chadha V, Lockington D, Kemp EG. Topical mitomycin C chemotherapy in the management of ocular surface neoplasia: a 10-year review of treatment outcomes and complications. Br J Ophthalmol. 2010;94(10):1316–21.

13. Ramasubramanian A, Shields CL, Sinha N, Shields JA. Ocular surface squamous neoplasia after corneal graft. Am J Ophthalmol. 2010;149(1):62–5.

14. Wilson MW, Hungerford JL, George SM, et al. Topical mitomycin C for the treatment of conjunctival and corneal epithelial dysplasia and neoplasia. Am J Ophthalmol. 1997;124:303–11.

15. Frucht-Pery J, Rozenman Y, Pe'er J. Topical mitomycin-C for partially excised conjunctival squamous cell carcinoma. Ophthalmology. 2002;109:548–52.

16. Shields CL, Naseripour M, Shields JA, et al. Topical mitomycin C for extensive, recurrent conjunctival-corneal squamous cell carcinoma. Am J Ophthalmol. 2002;133:601–6.

17. Chen C, Louis D, Dodd T, et al. Mitomycin C as an adjunct in the treatment of localised ocular surface squamous neoplasia. Br J Ophthalmol. 2004;88:17–8.

18. Birkholz ES, Goins KM, Sutphin JE, Kitzmann AS, Wagoner MD. Treatment of ocular surface squamous cell intraepithelial neoplasia with and without mitomycin C. Cornea. 2011;30(1):37–41.

19. Rudkin AK, Dempster L, Muecke JS. Management of diffuse ocular surface squamous neoplasia: efficacy and complications of topical chemotherapy. Clin Exp Ophthalmol. 2015;43(1):20–5.

20. Özcan AA, Çiloğlu E, Esen E, Şimdivar GH. Use of topical bevacizumab for conjunctival intraepithelial neoplasia. Cornea. 2014;33:1205–9.

21. McKelvie PA, Daniell M. Impression cytology following mitomycin C therapy for ocular surface squamous neoplasia. Br J Ophthalmol. 2001;85:1115–9.

22. de Keizer RJW, de Wolff-Rouendall D, van Delft JL. Topical application of 5-fluorouracil in premalignant lesions of cornea, conjunctiva and eyelid. Doc Ophthalmol. 1986;64:31–42.

23. Yeatts RP, Engelbrecht NE, Curry CD, et al. 5-Fluorouracil for the treatment of intraepithelial neoplasia of the conjunctiva and cornea. Ophthalmology. 2000;107:2190–5.

24. Yeatts RP, Ford JG, Stanton CA, et al. Topical 5-fluorouracil in treating epithelial neoplasia of the conjunctival and cornea. Ophthalmology. 1995;102:1338–44.

25. Midena E, Degli Angeli C, Valenti M, de Belvis V, Boccato P. Treatment of conjunctival squamous cell carcinoma with topical 5-fluorouracil. Br J Ophthalmol. 2000;84:268–72.

26. Rudkin AK, Muecke JS. Adjuvant 5-fluorouracil in the treatment of localised ocular surface squamous neoplasia. Br J Ophthalmol. 2011;95:947–50.

27. Parrozzani R, Frizziero L, Trainiti S, et al. Topical 1% 5-fluorouracil as a sole treatment of corneoconjunctival ocular surface squamous neoplasia: long-term study. Br J Ophthalmol. 2017;101:1094–9.

28. Parrozzani R, Lazzarini D, Alemany-Rubio E, et al. Topical 1% 5-fluorouracil in ocular surface squamous neoplasia: a long-term safety study. Br J Ophthalmol. 2011;95:355–9. https://doi.org/10.1136/bjo.2010.183244.

29. Joag MG, Sise A, Murillo JC, et al. Topical 5-fluorouracil 1% as primary treatment for ocular surface squamous neoplasia. Ophthalmology. 2016;123(7):1442–8.

30. Maskin SL. Regression of limbal epithelial dysplasia with topical interferon. Arch Ophthalmol. 1994;112:1145–6.

31. Kim J, Modlin RL, Moy RL, Dubinett SM, McHugh T, Nickoloff BJ, Uyemura K. IL-10 production in cutaneous basal and squamous cell carcinomas. A mechanism for evading the local T cell immune response. J Immunol. 1995;155(4):2240–7.

32. Karp CL, Galor A, Chhabra S, Barnes SD, Alfonso EC. Subconjunctival/perilesional recombinant interferon α2b for ocular surface squamous neoplasia: a 10-year review. Ophthalmology. 2010;117(12):2241–6.

33. Vann RR, Karp CL. Perilesional and topical interferon alfa-2b for conjunctival and corneal neoplasia. Ophthalmology. 1999;106:91–7.

34. Karp CL, Moore JK, Rosa RH. Treatment of conjunctival and corneal intraepithelial neoplasia with topical interferon alpha-2b. Ophthalmology. 2001;108:1093–8.

35. Boehm MD, Huang AJ. Treatment of recurrent corneal and conjunctival intraepithelial neoplasia with topical interferon alpha-2b. Ophthalmology. 2004;111:1755–61.
36. Galor A, Karp CL, Chhabra S, et al. Topical interferon alpha 2b eye-drops for treatment of ocular surface squamous neoplasia: a dose comparison study. Br J Ophthalmol. 2010;94:551–4.
37. Schechter BA, Koreishi AF, Karp CL, Feuer W. Long-term follow-up of conjunctival and corneal intraepithelial neoplasia treated with topical interferon alfa-2b. Ophthalmology. 2008;115:1291–l6.
38. Nanji AA, Sayyad FE, Karp CL. Topical chemotherapy for ocular surface squamous neoplasia. Curr Opin Ophthalmol. 2013;24:336–42.
39. Faramarzi A, Feizi S. Subconjunctival bevacizumab injection for ocular surface squamous neoplasia. Cornea. 2013;32:998–1001.
40. Paul S, Stone DU. Intralesional bevacizumab use for invasive ocular surface squamous neoplasia. J Ocul Pharmacol Ther. 2012;28:647–9.
41. Asena L, Dursun Altinors D. Topical Nevacizumab for the treatment of ocular surface squamous neoplasia. J Ocul Pharmacol Ther. 2015;31(8):487–90.
42. Finger PT, Chin KJ. Refractory squamous cell carcinoma of the conjunctiva treated with subconjunctival ranibizumab (Lucentis): a two-year study. Ophthal Plast Reconstr Surg. 2012;28:85–9.
43. Adler E, Turner JR, Stone DU. Ocular surface squamous neoplasia: a survey of changes in the standard of care from 2003 to 2012. Cornea. 2013;32:1558–61.
44. Arepalli S, Kaliki S, Shields CL, et al. Plaque radiotherapy in the management of scleral-invasive conjunctival squamous cell carcinoma: an analysis of 15 eyes. JAMA Ophthalmol. 2014;132:691–6.
45. Shields JA, Shields CL, DePotter P. Surgical management of conjunctival tumors. Arch Ophthalmol. 1997;115:808–15.
46. Sudesh S, Rapuano CJ, Cohen EJ, Eagle RC Jr, Laibson PR. Surgical management of ocular surface squamous neoplasms: the experience from a cornea center. Cornea. 2000;19(3):278–83.
47. Palamar M, Kaya E, Egrilmez S, Akalin T, Yagci A. Amniotic membrane transplantation in surgical management of ocular surface squamous neoplasias: long-term results. Eye. 2014;28(9):1131–5.
48. Cha SB, Shields CL, Shields JA, Eagel RC Jr, De Potter P, Talansky M. Massive precorneal extension of squamous cell carcinoma of the conjunctiva. Cornea. 1993;12(6):537–40.
49. Pizzarello LD, Jacobiec FA. Bowen's disease of the conjunctiva: a misnomer. In: Jacobiec FA, editor. Ocular and adnexal tumors. Birmingham, AL: Aesculapius; 1978. p. 553–71.
50. Erie JC, Campbell RJ, Liesegang TJ. Conjunctival and corneal intraepithelial and invasive neoplasia. Ophthalmology. 1986;93:176–83.
51. Li AS, et al. Recurrence of ocular surface squamous neoplasia treated with excisional biopsy and cryotherapy. Am J Ophthalmol. 2015;160(2):213–219.e1.
52. Siedlecki AN, Tapp S, Tosteson ANA, et al. Surgical versus interferon alpha-2b treatment strategies for ocular surface squamous neoplasia: a literature-based decision analysis. Cornea. 2016;35(5):613–8.
53. Tabin G, Levin S, Snibson G, et al. Late recurrences and the necessity for long-term follow-up in corneal and conjunctival intraepithelial neoplasia. Ophthalmology. 1997;104:485–92.
54. Philipp W, Daxecker F, Langmayr J, Gottinger W. Spontaneous corneal rupture after strontium irradiation of a conjunctival squamous cell carcinoma. Ophthalmologica. 1987;195:113–8.
55. Lommatzsch P. Beta-ray treatment of malignant epithelial tumors of the conjunctiva. Am J Ophthalmol. 1976;81:198–206.
56. Kearsley JH, Fitchew RS, Taylor RG. Adjunctive radiotherapy with strontium-90 in the treatment of conjunctival squamous cell carcinoma. Int J Radiat Oncol Biol Phys. 1988;14(3):435–43.
57. Lui H, Hobbs L, Tope WD, Lee PK, Elmets C, Provost N, Chan A, Neyndorff H, Su XY, Jain H, Hamzavi I, McLean D, Bissonnette R. Photodynamic therapy of multiple nonmelanoma skin cancers with verteporfin and red light-emitting diodes: two-year results evaluating tumor response and cosmetic outcomes. Arch Dermatol. 2004;140(1):26–32.
58. Barbazetto IA, Lee TC, Abramson DH. Treatment of conjunctival squamous cell carcinoma with photodynamic therapy. Am J Ophthalmol. 2004;138(2):183–9.

Intraocular Lymphoma

George N. Magrath and Emil Anthony T. Say

Introduction

Lymphoma is a rare ocular malignancy affecting a myriad of intraocular structures, each with unique clinical features [1]. Although diagnosis may sometimes be challenging, early recognition and initiation of treatment are critical because of potential systemic and central nervous system (CNS) involvement.

Intraocular lymphoma represents less than 1% of all extranodal non-Hodgkin's lymphoma. It is easiest to understand by differentiating whether there is vitreoretinal or uveal involvement. Vitreoretinal lymphoma (VRL) is highly associated with CNS lymphoma [2]. On the contrary, majority of uveal lymphomas (UL) have isolated ocular disease [2]. Localization of lymphoma within the eye guides systemic evaluation and treatment, and determines patient prognosis.

Vitreoretinal Lymphoma

VRL was first described in 1951 [3] and is the more common form of intraocular lymphoma. It mainly affects the elderly, often between 50 and 60 years of age, but may affect younger patients who are immunosuppressed. Bilateral disease is noted in 40% of cases [4], and 80% will have either sequential or simultaneous CNS lymphoma [1]. Although primary VRL with or without CNS involvement is the most well-described and frequent presentation, there have been recent reports of secondary (metastatic) VRL from systemic non-Hodgkin's lymphoma, with some estimating that 5% of all VRL are secondary [5]. Nevertheless, the vast majority of VRL will still be categorized as diffuse large B-cell lymphoma (DLBCL), whether they are primary or secondary (metastatic) [5–7] (Table 1).

G. N. Magrath · E. A. T. Say (✉)
Storm Eye Institute, Medical University of South Carolina, Charleston, SC, USA

© Springer Nature Singapore Pte Ltd. 2019
A. Ramasubramanian (ed.), *Ocular Oncology*, Current Practices in
Ophthalmology, https://doi.org/10.1007/978-981-13-7538-5_6

Table 1 Intraocular lymphoma

	Vitreoretinal lymphoma	Uveal lymphoma
Age	Usually >60 years old	Usually >60 years old
Clinical features	– Mostly bilateral – CNS involvement – Vitreous haze/vitritis – Multifocal sub-RPE infiltrate	– Unilateral or bilateral – Ocular adnexal involvement – Patchy or diffuse choroidal infiltrate with extra scleral extension
Lymphoma subtype	**Primary:** Diffuse large B-cell lymphoma **Secondary:** Diffuse large B-cell lymphoma	**Primary:** Extranodal marginal zone lymphoma **Secondary:** Diffuse large B-cell lymphoma
Ultrasound	Vitreous opacities and normal choroid	Choroidal thickening and extrascleral extension with low internal reflectivity
Fundus autofluorescence	"Leopard-spot pattern"	Mixed hyper- and hypoautofluorescence
Fluorescein angiography	Mixed hyper and hypofluorescence	Mixed hyper and hypofluorescence
Indocyanine green angiography	Hypofluorescent infiltrates	Hypofluorescent infiltrates
EDI-OCT	Multifocal pigment epithelial detachments, vitreous opacities, subretinal infiltrates	Undulating or "seasick" contour and thickened choroid

CNS central nervous system, RPE retinal pigment epithelium, EDI-OCT enhanced depth imaging optical coherence tomography
Differential demographic, clinical, and imaging features of vitreoretinal and uveal lymphoma

Clinical Appearance

Generally, VRL is the occurrence of vitritis in patients not otherwise expected to mount a vigorous inflammatory response in the vitreous, such as the elderly or the immunosuppressed. By ophthalmoscopy, the accumulation of subretinal and sub-retinal pigment epithelial (RPE) deposits of lymphocytes can masquerade as various forms of uveitis (Fig. 1). In 1984 Gass et al. [8] provided a concise description of the vitritis with sub-RPE deposits that occurs frequently in VRL. The initial accumulation of lymphocytes often occurs in a perivascular pattern, mimicking a vasculitis, followed by numerous cream-colored peripheral sub-RPE deposits that simulate white dot syndromes. As these lesions coalesce, larger areas of cream-colored subretinal and sub-RPE infiltrates can form that may be similar to acute retinal necrosis or metastatic tumors. Further accumulation of these infiltrates can lead to areas of increased pigmentation. Retinal involvement typically occurs in the equatorial region, but optic nerve or macular involvement can sometimes be seen. Occasionally, spontaneous regression, even without treatment, may occur in vitreoretinal lymphoma leading to delays in diagnosis. It is also worthwhile to discuss a rare presentation of a transient vitelliform submaculopathy that occurs as a paraneoplastic response preceding the diagnosis of primary VRL or CNS lymphoma [9].

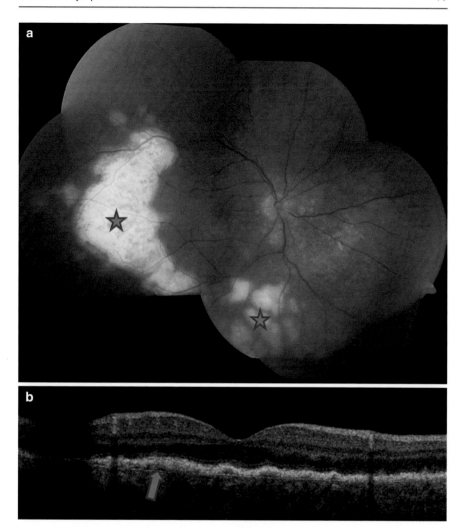

Fig. 1 Primary vitreoretinal lymphoma. (**a**) Fundus photograph of the right eye revealing multifocal creamy, yellow lesions at the level of the subretinal and sub-RPE space (asterisk). (**b**) OCT through the macula confirming the infiltrate at the level of the subretinal and sub-RPE space (arrow)

Vitreous involvement occurs as discreet, homogenous, suspended cells with a general haze within the vitreous cavity. The cells generally do not clump into clusters, and appear to line along vitreous fibrils, producing an "aurora borealis" appearance behind the lens on slit-lamp biomicroscopy [2]. It represents both a reactive inflammatory response with macrophages and the lymphomatous clonal population. This composition of inflammatory cells, macrophages, and lymphoma cells can mimic vitritis from posterior uveitis. Telling clues that vitritis is secondary to lymphoma, and not inflammatory in origin, include the absence of cystoid macular edema, a relatively preserved vitreous structure, and a lack of durable response to steroids.

Other uncommon clinical features of VRL include retinal vascular occlusions, nerve fiber layer infarcts, hemorrhages, and iris neovascularization, all of which could result in significant visual compromise. However, it is still the combination of vitritis and sub-RPE infiltrates with or without subretinal and intraretinal infiltration in elderly patients that most consider hallmarks of VRL, and which will allow differentiation from masquerades.

Imaging Features of Vitreoretinal Lymphoma

Advances in imaging modalities have made dramatic improvements in diagnosis of VRL. Autofluorescence can reveal granular hyper- and hypo-autofluorescence consistent with sub-RPE involvement initially ("leopard-spot pattern"), while intravenous fluorescein angiography shows hyper- and hypofluorescent lesions in reverse of autofluorescence [10]. Indocyanine green is generally nondiagnostic, but may show hypofluorescent infiltrates [11]. Enhanced depth imaging-optical coherence tomography (EDI-OCT) is particularly useful in disease localization, and often will show hyperreflective infiltrates in the sub-RPE, subretinal, and intraretinal space in decreasing frequency, as well as vitreous cells [12].

Diagnosis

Despite advances in retinal imaging, cytopathologic confirmation remains the gold standard in diagnosis of VRL. However, in the presence of known CNS lymphoma and typical clinical features, diagnosis of VRL can be made presumptively. In atypical cases, a vitreous biopsy by pars plana vitrectomy with or without chorioretinal biopsy can be very helpful [13]. It should be emphasized that lymphoma cells tend to be very fragile and will lyse without purposeful care. Additionally, there may also be a significant background of infiltrative inflammatory cells and macrophages, which can cloud the diagnosis for pathologists not accustomed to eye samples. A strong collaboration between the ophthalmologist and pathologist is crucial in obtaining a robust result from each biopsy. Flow cytometry allows further identification of clonal populations of lymphocytes. It should be noted that in general, the diagnostic yield of vitreous biopsies is low in cases wherein malignancy is suspected. In fact, among eyes undergoing diagnostic vitrectomy, there is a significantly less yield in eyes suspected to have malignancy compared to those suspected to have an underlying infection (10% vs. 42%, $p = 0.02$) [13]. Given the diagnostic dilemmas that may occur in cases where malignancy is suspected but cytopathology is equivocal, several surrogate tests have been reported. These include IL-10/IL-6 ratios, IgH gene rearrangement, chemokine and chemokine receptor expression, as well as MyD88 testing [14, 15]. Currently, the clinical utility of these tests is still under debate and they do not replace cytopathology as the gold standard.

Patients with VRL should routinely receive imaging of the brain and spine, in conjunction with a neuro-oncologist. These patients should receive neurological examinations to identify any focal deficits. Screening should continue for an extended amount of time as CNS lymphoma is closely related to VRL. Despite recent reports of secondary VRL, it is still unknown whether routine systemic evaluation should be performed in patients diagnosed with VRL without known CNS or systemic lymphoma.

Treatment

There is currently no consensus on preferred method of local therapy in eyes with VRL. Further, the precise role of systemic therapy in patients presenting with VRL without CNS lymphoma is still undetermined. Given these uncertainties, current recommendations by a panel of worldwide experts from the primary CNS lymphoma collaborative group symposium include the following [2]:

1. For VRL without CNS involvement, local therapy either with intravitreal chemotherapy or external beam radiation (EBRT) is still preferred regardless of laterality, although systemic treatment should not be completely excluded.
2. For VRL with concurrent CNS involvement, either high-dose methotrexate-based systemic chemotherapy in conjunction with local intravitreal chemotherapy or whole-brain radiotherapy with ocular radiotherapy is recommended.

The role of systemic chemotherapy as prophylaxis against future development of CNS lymphoma is still under debate. Currently available literature is limited by small case series, variations in treatment strategies, and lack of prospective trials. Perhaps one of the biggest developments would come from a 17-center European collaborative study wherein 78 patients with only PVRL without CNS lymphoma were grouped according to treatment regimen (ocular therapy, systemic chemotherapy, or both). Overall, 36% developed CNS lymphoma at a median follow-up of 49 months. More importantly, there was no significant difference in the occurrence of CNS lymphoma across the three groups, but 23% of patients receiving systemic chemotherapy developed severe adverse events, most commonly acute renal failure [16].

Regarding local therapy, EBRT has been the traditional treatment method, whereas intravitreal chemotherapy with methotrexate, rituximab, and more recently melphalan has been more recently developed with equal success in tumor control [17–19].

EBRT is typically delivered in low doses (3000–3500 cGy) over several fractionations, allowing the patient to achieve complete treatment within a month. EBRT may also be combined with whole-brain radiation in patients with simultaneous CNS involvement [20]. Although radiation has excellent local control and is minimally invasive, potential complications include keratopathy, cataracts, radiation retinopathy, macular edema, and optic neuropathy. These complications may be vision threatening and may be difficult to treat [21]. Some experts even recommend that EBRT be always performed in both eyes, even in patients with unilateral involvement, as VRL will almost certainly develop bilateral disease [2].

The use of intravitreal chemotherapy has gained popularity in recent years, with methotrexate being the most popular. A protocol of 400 micrograms of methotrexate twice weekly during a 1-month induction, followed by weekly therapy, has excellent success in achieving remission of the disease typically within 13 injections but requiring extended monthly maintenance therapy [22–25]. There are significant local toxicities possible with intravitreal methotrexate including maculopathy, keratopathy, and progression of cataract. Recent experience with the biologic, rituximab, a humanized monoclonal antibody targeting CD20-positive B cells, has been encouraging [26]. The rise in the use of intravitreal melphalan for retinoblastoma has now translated to the use for VRL; however, its optimal dosage and frequency are still unknown. The use of intravitreal chemotherapy or biologic therapy provides a realistic alternative for either primary or secondary treatment of VRL.

Uveal Lymphoma

Similar to VRL, UL is also a disease of the elderly with a mean age of presentation at 62 years but is less frequent than VRL [1, 27]. In addition, they are also more indolent and low grade, with extranodal marginal zone lymphoma (EMZL) being the predominant type, seen in up to 80% [28]. At presentation, disease is often primary (69–77%), with only a few patients having associated systemic lymphoma metastatic to the uvea (secondary) [27, 28]. Although majority of patients achieve complete remission with treatment, UL often masquerades as other inflammatory or neoplastic diseases leading to misdiagnosis and treatment delays [28] (Table 1).

Clinical Appearance

Unlike VRL, bilateral involvement is not the rule in UL, with about half of cases being unilateral [27, 28]. Further, co-involvement of the ocular adnexa is frequent and seen in up to 60% of eyes, which could involve the orbit and/or conjunctiva [28]. Hence, a thorough slit-lamp and dilated fundus examination should be performed in patients with orbital or conjunctival lymphoma for accurate staging.

Choroidal lymphoma is the most frequent type of UL, comprising over 95% of cases [28]. It typically appears as multifocal patchy or confluent yellowish-white choroidal infiltrates on indirect ophthalmoscopy, which become more apparent with increasing thickness and may be associated with pigment clumping or serous retinal detachments, leading to decreased visual acuity. Choroidal folds are also visualized in up to 41% of cases [27] and rarely optic nerve infiltration can be a presenting sign [29]. Characteristically, choroidal lymphoma is painless, unlike posterior scleritis. The vitreous is mostly clear, and its clinical appearance often mimics white dot syndromes such as birdshot chorioretinopathy.

Iris and ciliary body infiltration is exceedingly rare and is often associated with more aggressive types of systemic lymphoma [27]. Irido-ciliary lymphoma often presents as a discrete white mass at either iris, angle, or ciliary body. Anterior chamber cells are frequently seen, very much similar to anterior uveitis in many cases. There may also be anisocoria, hyphema, pseudohypopyon, and ill-defined precipitates on the iris surface or endothelium. These patients may present with eye pain, unlike choroidal lymphoma, and many have decreased vision [1, 30, 31]. Given that most irido-ciliary lymphomas are more aggressive types of lymphoma, they also have worse life prognosis [32].

Imaging Features of Uveal Lymphoma

Ancillary testing is vastly different in UL compared to VRL. In the former, evaluation with ultrasonography (76%), orbital MRI (70%), or CT scan (57%), in decreasing significance of detecting extrascleral extension, is of utmost importance to determine the extent of involvement [28]. By ultrasonography, choroidal thickening with or without subretinal fluid is the characteristic finding and reveals low internal reflectivity whether it is irido-ciliary or choroidal. Extra scleral extension is often adjacent to choroidal thickening and has low internal reflectivity as well [33]. Fundus autofluorescence is often unrevealing, with multifocal choroidal infiltrates being slightly hyperautofluorescent and confluent lesions often have a mixed hyper- and hypoautofluorescent components, especially when pigment clumping is visible [34]. Infiltrates generally manifest blocked fluorescence in both fluorescein and indocyanine green angiography but are more readily visible with the latter [28]. EDI-OCT reveals choroidal thickening with loss of normal choroidal details and a rippled RPE-Bruch's membrane layer giving a characteristic "seasick" undulating appearance [35].

Diagnosis

Histopathologic confirmation is still the gold standard for UL; however, given its high extraocular involvement, tissue samples are more readily available compared to VRL. When systemic or ocular adnexal involvement is detected simultaneously, peripheral lymph node or adnexal tissue biopsies can be performed; however, if only intraocular involvement is present, transvitreal or transscleral fine-needle aspiration biopsy or pars plana vitrectomy with chorioretinal biopsy is the valid option [27, 28]. Given its greater access to tissue samples, diagnostic yield is generally better than VRL.

Although there is consensus that EMZL is most frequent, other less common types include follicular cell lymphoma, DLBCL, multiple myeloma, human T-cell leukemia virus lymphoma, and human acquired immune deficiency syndrome-associated lymphoma [27, 28, 32, 36]. Benign reactive lymphoid hyperplasia has previously been used to describe histopathologic features in some cases, but with current immunohistochemical and polymerase chain reaction testing re-evaluation often reveals that up to 80% can now be reclassified as malignant non-Hodgkin's lymphoma [37].

Treatment

At the time of diagnosis, systemic staging is important, as about 20% will have coexisting systemic disease with workup, especially if there is bilateral involvement [27, 28]. In terms of survival, primary UL without systemic involvement has better prognosis with no lymphoma-related deaths versus 33% lymphoma-related deaths for secondary UL in one series [27]. In addition, younger patients should be assessed for immunodeficiency.

Management strategies for UL are similar to VRL, but a standard optimal treatment algorithm has not been established. For isolated ocular disease, especially when unilateral, most centers prefer low-dose EBRT. This typically induces complete regression in almost all cases with few side effects [38]. Radiation dose also varies according to histologic subtype, varying from 2800 to 4000 cGy. In patients with bilateral involvement or with coexisting active systemic disease, systemic chemotherapy with single agent rituximab, or combination therapy for more aggressive disease, may be necessary.

Overall, complete remission is achieved in about 80% of cases [28]. Further, those with localized ocular disease rarely develop relapse [27, 28]. Despite these favorable results, continued systemic evaluation should still be performed.

Summary

Intraocular lymphomas are rare malignancies that can be classified either as VRL or as UL, each with distinct clinical appearance, pathologic features, and systemic prognosis. VRL generally presents with bilateral vitreoretinal infiltrates, associated CNS involvement, and poor life prognosis, while UL often presents with patchy or diffuse choroidal infiltration, and associated ocular adnexal involvement, but infrequent systemic disease, and hence a better life prognosis. Both types of lymphoma typically occur in the elderly and can masquerade as various inflammatory or infectious conditions; thus, a high index of suspicion is necessary to avoid delays in diagnosis and initiation of proper therapy.

References

1. Coupland SE, Damato B. Understanding intraocular lymphomas. Clin Exp Ophthalmol. 2008;36(6):564–78.
2. Chan CC, Rubenstein JL, Coupland SE, Davis JL, Harbour JW, Johnston PB, et al. Primary vitreoretinal lymphoma: a report from an International Primary Central Nervous System Lymphoma Collaborative Group symposium. Oncologist. 2011;16(11):1589–99.

3. Cooper EL, Riker JL. Malignant lymphoma of the uveal tract. Am J Ophthalmol. 1951;34(8):1153–8.

4. Levasseur SD, Wittenberg LA, White VA. Vitreoretinal lymphoma: a 20-year review of incidence, clinical and cytologic features, treatment, and outcomes. JAMA Ophthalmol. 2013;131(1):50–5.

5. Salomao DR, Pulido JS, Johnston PB, Canal-Fontcuberta I, Feldman AL. Vitreoretinal presentation of secondary large B-cell lymphoma in patients with systemic lymphoma. JAMA Ophthalmol. 2013;131(9):1151–8.

6. Cao X, Shen D, Callanan DG, Mochizuki M, Chan CC. Diagnosis of systemic metastatic retinal lymphoma. Acta Ophthalmol. 2011;89(2):e149–54.

7. Taki R, Takeda A, Yoshikawa H, Fukuhara T, Arita R, Suehiro Y, et al. Clinical features of systemic metastatic retinal lymphoma in Japanese patients. Ocul Immunol Inflamm. 2017;25(5):654–62.

8. Gass JD, Sever RJ, Grizzard WS, Clarkson JG, Blumenkranz M, Wind CA, et al. Multifocal pigment epithelial detachments by reticulum cell sarcoma. A characteristic funduscopic picture. Retina. 1984;4(3):135–43.

9. Pang CE, Shields CL, Jumper JM, Yannuzzi LA. Paraneoplastic cloudy vitelliform submaculopathy in primary vitreoretinal lymphoma. Am J Ophthalmol. 2014;158(6):1253–61.e2.

10. Casady M, Faia L, Nazemzadeh M, Nussenblatt R, Chan CC, Sen HN. Fundus autofluorescence patterns in primary intraocular lymphoma. Retina. 2014;34(2):366–72.

11. Fardeau C, Lee CP, Merle-Beral H, Cassoux N, Bodaghi B, Davi F, et al. Retinal fluorescein, indocyanine green angiography, and optic coherence tomography in non-Hodgkin primary intraocular lymphoma. Am J Ophthalmol. 2009;147(5):886–94. 94.e1.

12. Barry RJ, Tasiopoulou A, Murray PI, Patel PJ, Sagoo MS, Denniston AK, et al. Characteristic optical coherence tomography findings in patients with primary vitreoretinal lymphoma: a novel aid to early diagnosis. Br J Ophthalmol. 2018;102(10):1362–6.

13. Mruthyunjaya P, Jumper JM, McCallum R, Patel DJ, Cox TA, Jaffe GJ. Diagnostic yield of vitrectomy in eyes with suspected posterior segment infection or malignancy. Ophthalmology. 2002;109(6):1123–9.

14. Chan CC. Molecular pathology of primary intraocular lymphoma. Trans Am Ophthalmol Soc. 2003;101:275–92.

15. Pulido JS, Salomao DR, Frederick LA, Viswanatha DS. MyD-88 L265P mutations are present in some cases of vitreoretinal lymphoma. Retina. 2015;35(4):624–7.

16. Riemens A, Bromberg J, Touitou V, Sobolewska B, Missotten T, Baarsma S, et al. Treatment strategies in primary vitreoretinal lymphoma: a 17-center European collaborative study. JAMA Ophthalmol. 2015;133(2):191–7.

17. Chan CC, Sen HN. Current concepts in diagnosing and managing primary vitreoretinal (intraocular) lymphoma. Discov Med. 2013;15(81):93–100.

18. Pe'er J, Hochberg FH, Foster CS. Clinical review: treatment of vitreoretinal lymphoma. Ocul Immunol Inflamm. 2009;17(5):299–306.

19. Shields CL, Sioufi K, Mashayekhi A, Shields JA. Intravitreal melphalan for treatment of primary vitreoretinal lymphoma: a new indication for an old drug. JAMA Ophthalmol. 2017;135(7):815–8.

20. Berenbom A, Davila RM, Lin HS, Harbour JW. Treatment outcomes for primary intraocular lymphoma: implications for external beam radiotherapy. Eye (Lond). 2007;21(9):1198–201.

21. Hoffman PM, McKelvie P, Hall AJ, Stawell RJ, Santamaria JD. Intraocular lymphoma: a series of 14 patients with clinicopathological features and treatment outcomes. Eye (Lond). 2003;17(4):513–21.

22. Fishburne BC, Wilson DJ, Rosenbaum JT, Neuwelt EA. Intravitreal methotrexate as an adjunctive treatment of intraocular lymphoma. Arch Ophthalmol. 1997;115(9):1152–6.

23. Smith JR, Rosenbaum JT, Wilson DJ, Doolittle ND, Siegal T, Neuwelt EA, et al. Role of intravitreal methotrexate in the management of primary central nervous system lymphoma with ocular involvement. Ophthalmology. 2002;109(9):1709–16.

24. Frenkel S, Hendler K, Siegal T, Shalom E, Pe'er J. Intravitreal methotrexate for treating vitreo-retinal lymphoma: 10 years of experience. Br J Ophthalmol. 2008;92(3):383–8.
25. de Smet MD. Management of non Hodgkin's intraocular lymphoma with intravitreal metho-trexate. Bull Soc Belge Ophtalmol. 2001;279:91–5.
26. Kitzmann AS, Pulido JS, Mohney BG, Baratz KH, Grube T, Marler RJ, et al. Intraocular use of rituximab. Eye (Lond). 2007;21(12):1524–7.
27. Mashayekhi A, Shukla SY, Shields JA, Shields CL. Choroidal lymphoma: clinical features and association with systemic lymphoma. Ophthalmology. 2014;121(1):342–51.
28. Aronow ME, Portell CA, Sweetenham JW, Singh AD. Uveal lymphoma: clinical features, diagnostic studies, treatment selection, and outcomes. Ophthalmology. 2014;121(1):334–41.
29. Tavallali A, Shields CL, Bianciotto C, Shields JA. Choroidal lymphoma masquerading as ante-rior ischemic optic neuropathy. Eur J Ophthalmol. 2010;20(5):959–62.
30. Pelegrin L, Adan A, Lopez-Guillermo A, Martinez A, Shields CL. An old disease in an atypical place. Surv Ophthalmol. 2014;59(6):660–3.
31. Velez G, de Smet MD, Whitcup SM, Robinson M, Nussenblatt RB, Chan CC. Iris involve-ment in primary intraocular lymphoma: report of two cases and review of the literature. Surv Ophthalmol. 2000;44(6):518–26.
32. Mashayekhi A, Shields CL, Shields JA. Iris involvement by lymphoma: a review of 13 cases. Clin Exp Ophthalmol. 2013;41(1):19–26.
33. Chang TS, Byrne SF, Gass JD, Hughes JR, Johnson RN, Murray TG. Echographic findings in benign reactive lymphoid hyperplasia of the choroid. Arch Ophthalmol. 1996;114(6):669–75.
34. Schubert CGAS, Shields CL. The seasick pattern of choroidal lymphoma on enhanced depth imaging optical coherence tomography. Retina. 2014;34(8):1495–512.
35. Shields CL, Arepalli S, Pellegrini M, Mashayekhi A, Shields JA. Choroidal lymphoma shows calm, rippled, or undulating topography on enhanced depth imaging optical coherence tomog-raphy in 14 eyes. Retina. 2014;34(7):1347–53.
36. Grossniklaus HE, Martin DF, Avery R, Shields JA, Shields CL, Kuo IC, et al. Uveal lym-phoid infiltration: report of four cases and clinicopathologic review. Ophthalmology. 1998;105(7):1265–73.
37. Cockerham GC, Hidayat AA, Bijwaard KE, Sheng ZM. Re-evaluation of "reactive lym-phoid hyperplasia of the uvea": an immunohistochemical and molecular analysis of 10 cases. Ophthalmology. 2000;107(1):151–8.
38. Mashayekhi A, Hasanreisoglu M, Shields CL, Shields JA. External beam radiation for choroi-dal lymphoma: efficacy and complications. Retina. 2016;36(10):2006–12.

Update on Management of Coats' Disease

Janelle Fassbender Adeniran, Oluwasayo Akinyosoye, and Aparna Ramasubramanian

Introduction

Definition and General Statements Regarding Coats' Disease

(a) Definition: Coats' disease is an exudative retinopathy characterized by light-bulb aneurysms, capillary non-perfusion, progression to exudative retinal detachment, and, if untreated, neovascular glaucoma and phthisis bulbi [1].

(b) Epidemiology: Coats' disease is an exudative retinopathy characterized by light-bulb aneurysms and capillary non-perfusion with progression to exudative retinal detachment and, if untreated, neovascular glaucoma and phthisis bulbi. It is typically a unilateral disease affecting boys and girls in a 3:1 ratio with an average age of onset between 8 and 16 years [2]. Despite the average age, new-onset Coats' disease of adults into their eighth decade is reported in the literature [3]. Treatment strategies vary and include cryotherapy, laser photocoagulation, external drainage of subretinal fluid, scleral buckling, and pars plana vitrectomy [4]. Adjunctive intravitreal injection of corticosteroids [5, 6] and, more recently, anti-vascular endothelial growth factor (VEGF) have also been implemented [7–9]. Treatment is individualized based on presenting symptoms and progression of disease.

(c) Histopathology: Subretinal exudation associated with dilated and telangiectatic vessels results in deposition of cholesterol and foamy histiocytes that variably cause thickening of the outer retina [10].

J. F. Adeniran · O. Akinyosoye · A. Ramasubramanian (✉)
Department of Ophthalmology and Visual Sciences, University of Louisville, Louisville, KY, USA
e-mail: aparna.ramasubramanian@louisville.edu

© Springer Nature Singapore Pte Ltd. 2019
A. Ramasubramanian (ed.), *Ocular Oncology*, Current Practices in Ophthalmology, https://doi.org/10.1007/978-981-13-7538-5_7

Clinical Presentation

(a) Patients with Coats' disease may present in a variety of ways depending on the area affected by the retinal telangiectasia and exudation. Unilateral vision loss occurs with exudation affecting the macula but patients may be incidentally noted to have peripheral telangiectasia with or without exudation. Advanced cases may present with heterochromia, leukocoria, strabismus, nystagmus, or pain from neovascular glaucoma [2]. Approximately 90% of eyes present with a normal anterior-segment exam but visual acuity may vary from 20/20 to no light perception [11]. Although classically Coats' disease is unilateral, reports utilizing newer, wide-field imaging modalities do note mild changes in the fellow eye. Moreover, symptomatic, bilateral disease is seen in systemic syndromes such as facioscapulohumeral dystrophy [12], Turner's syndrome [13], Senior-Loken syndrome [14], and Coats' plus disease [15]. In addition to retinal telangiectasia and intraretinal exudates, exam may show exudative retinal detachment, vasoproliferative tumor, or retinal microcyst. In cases with advanced ischemia, peripheral or optic disc neovascularization may occur but this is rare [16, 17]. Neovascular glaucoma leading to a blind, painful eye will likely lead to enucleation [1]. Some patients present with permanent vision loss due to macular fibrosis, which may, in some cases, be due to choroidal or retinal neovascularization [18, 19]. Epiretinal membrane may occur in 2–4% of patients and patients can do well with vitrectomy and membrane peeling [20, 21]. Coats' disease in adults has a slower progression of the disease with less severe features [22, 23]. The clinical course varies per patient but is generally slowly progressive and rarely has spontaneous remission [24].

(b) It is important, especially in advanced pediatric presentations of Coats' disease, that retinoblastoma be included in the differential. Additional diagnoses to consider include familial exudative vitreoretinopathy, persistent hyperplastic proliferative vitreoretinopathy, Norrie disease, or retinopathy of prematurity [25]. Diagnoses to consider in adult-onset Coats' disease include sarcoidosis, Eales' disease, choroidal hemangioma, tuberculosis, idiopathic retinal vasculitis aneurysms and neuroretinitis (IRVAN), or sickle-cell retinopathy [17].

Staging

(a) A staging classification devised by Shields et al. is as follows [10]:

Stage	Clinical findings
1	Retinal telangiectasia
2	Telangiectasia and exudates (a) Extrafoveal exudates (b) Foveal exudates

Stage	Clinical findings
3	Exudative retinal detachment
	(a) Subtotal detachment
	1. Extrafoveal
	2. Foveal
	(b) Total retinal detachment
4	Total retinal detachment and glaucoma
5	Advanced end-stage disease

Nonsurgical Management

Introduction

1. Treatment strategies vary and include cryotherapy, laser photocoagulation, external drainage of subretinal fluid, scleral buckling, and pars plana vitrectomy [4]. Adjunctive intravitreal injection of corticosteroids [5, 6] and, more recently, anti-vascular endothelial growth factor (VEGF) have also been implemented [7–9]. Treatment is individualized based on presenting symptoms and progression of disease, yet there have been no randomized, clinical trials to demonstrate efficacy of one modality over another. Moreover, the frequency of complications including vision-limiting vitreoretinal fibrosis, tractional retinal detachment (TRD), neovascular glaucoma, and enucleation is unknown, and their relation to individual treatment strategies is especially unclear.
2. The approach to management includes in-depth consultation with family members of the affected child. Risks of treatment include cataract, ocular inflammation, progressive exudative detachment, vitreoretinal fibrosis, choroidal detachment, rhegmatogenous retinal detachment, and hemorrhage. Observation is typical in late stages but if the disease progresses to neovascular glaucoma, a blind and painful eye may warrant enucleation. Alternatives to ablative treatment include intravitreal corticosteroids, intravitreal anti-vascular endothelial growth factor (anti-VEGF), and minimally invasive surgical procedures.

Ablative Therapies

1. Preoperative testing during exam under anesthesia allows for targeting of abnormal telangiectasias and capillary non-perfusion. Fluorescein angiography may be performed to aid both in diagnosis and in targeting treatment.
2. Laser photocoagulation: Most commonly argon green laser photocoagulation is used to treat areas of capillary non-perfusion and telangiectasia in the absence of exudative retinal detachment which may prevent adequate laser therapy [17]. However, reports have shown resolution of exudation via laser photocoagulation targeted to the telangiectatic vessels within the exudative detachment [26, 27]. Indirect laser is typically performed during EUA, but recent reports suggest

better visualization with two-port pars plana non-vitrectomy technique [28]. This is a more invasive approach and is not widely utilized at this time.

3. Cryotherapy: Cryotherapy is especially useful where extensive subretinal exudation precludes adequate laser photocoagulation. The minimum necessary cryoapplication can reduce the risk of subsequent patient discomfort, inflammation, cataract formation, and proliferative vitreoretinopathy (PVR) [17]. In more advanced cases, one report suggests that cryotherapy under air at the time of vitrectomy may minimize occurrence of PVR [29].
   (a) Technique: A double-freeze-thaw technique is utilized when applying cryotherapy. The sclera is indented transconjunctivally under a shallow exudative detachment until the probe is visualized [11]. The goal is to ablate the abnormal telangiectasias by direct visualization. Multiple sessions may be necessary and combined antibiotic and steroid ointment can be applied postoperatively to relieve ocular discomfort.

Pharmacologic Therapies

1. Steroids (triamcinolone acetonide) [6, 30] and off-label use of sustained-release dexamethasone (Ozurdex®) [5]:
   (a) Technique: Multiple techniques for injecting periocular triamcinolone acetonide (TA) can be utilized, including transseptal or posterior subtenon's capsule. Periocular administration avoids the potential complications of endophthalmitis (infectious or sterile) and iatrogenic retinal holes, especially in the presence of exudative retinal detachment. Intravitreal TA is typically delivered in 0.1 cc of 4 mg concentration. Patients should be monitored for ocular hypertension whether utilizing TA or a sustained-release intravitreal implant off-label.
2. Anti-VEGF agents including pegaptanib [31], bevacizumab [32–34], ranibizumab [35, 36], and aflibercept [37]:
   (a) Although many reports exist regarding the efficacy of anti-VEGF agents, questions remain regarding their mechanism of action and role in the pathogenesis vitreoretinal fibrosis. Although reports have shown elevated VEGF levels in the vitreous of Coats' patients [38], these are typically advanced cases where ischemia predominates. Furthermore, case series have shown that ablative therapy in addition to anti-VEGF may increase the risk of vitreoretinal fibrosis [35, 39]; however, other large series have not confirmed this occurrence [40]. These agents are also efficacious when used in combination with periocular or intravitreal steroids [9, 41].

Surgical Management

(a) Various vitreoretinal surgical techniques are employed in advanced Coats' disease where total or partial retinal detachment does not resolve with or precludes ablative or pharmacologic therapy.

1. External drainage of subretinal fluid is occasionally necessary to allow for effective laser photocoagulation or cryoapplication.
2. Management of retinal detachment with scleral buckle and external drainage of subretinal fluid may also be coupled with pars plana vitrectomy and gas endotamponade.

(b) Enucleation:

1. Indication for enucleation for Coats' disease includes a blind, painful eye that is typically the result of advanced neovascular glaucoma [11]. Around 5–16% of children receive enucleation as either initial management or disease progression as reported in the literature [11, 21]. Additionally, eyes may be enucleated if retinoblastoma cannot be excluded and a high suspicion remains [42].

Treatment Algorithm

(a) Treatment patterns vary according to institution and disease course but may be generalized by the following algorithm:

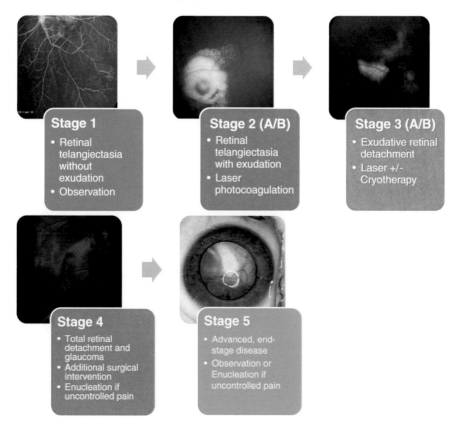

Pearls and Pitfalls

- Coats' disease is an exudative retinopathy characterized by retinal vascular abnormalities, light-bulb aneurysms, retinal telangiectasia, lipid exudates, and capillary non-perfusion which can progress to exudative retinal detachment.
- It is typically a unilateral disease affecting boys and girls in a 3:1 ratio with an average age of onset between 8 and 16 years.
- Although clinical presentation and progression are variable, patients commonly present with unilaterality, a normal anterior segment exam, and telangiectasia and intraretinal exudates on retinal exam.
- Coats' disease is rarely bilateral, and in children retinoblastoma must be ruled out.
- Treatment options include cryotherapy, laser photocoagulation, external drainage of subretinal fluid, scleral buckling, and pars plana vitrectomy and are individualized based on presenting symptoms and progression of disease:
  - Frequency of complications and its relationship to individual treatment strategies are unknown but include vitreoretinal fibrosis, tractional retinal detachment (TRD), neovascular glaucoma, and enucleation.

Conflict of Interest   None.

Funding Sources   This work was supported in part by an unrestricted institutional grant from Research to Prevent Blindness, NY, NY.

References

1. Shields JA, Shields CL. Review: Coats' disease: the 2001 LuEsther T. Mertz lecture. Retina. 2002;22(1):80–91.
2. Ghorbanian S, Jaulim A, Chatziralli IP. Diagnosis and treatment of Coats' disease: a review of the literature. Ophthalmologica. 2012;227(4):175–82.
3. Rishi E, et al. Coats' disease of adult-onset in 48 eyes. Indian J Ophthalmol. 2016;64(7): 518–23.
4. Sigler EJ, et al. Current management of Coats' disease. Surv Ophthalmol. 2014;59(1):30–46.
5. Saatci AO, Doruk HC, Yaman A. Intravitreal dexamethasone implant (Ozurdex) in Coats' disease. Case Rep Ophthalmol. 2013;4(3):122–8.
6. Ghazi NG, et al. Intravitreal triamcinolone in Coats' disease. Ophthalmology. 2012;119(3):648–9.
7. Chaudhary KM, Mititelu M, Lieberman RM. An evidence-based review of vascular endothelial growth factor inhibition in pediatric retinal diseases: part 2. Coats' disease, best disease, and uveitis with childhood neovascularization. J Pediatr Ophthalmol Strabismus. 2013;50(1):11–9.
8. Kaul S, et al. Intravitreal anti-vascular endothelial growth factor agents as an adjunct in the management of Coats' disease in children. Indian J Ophthalmol. 2010;58(1):76–8.
9. Cakir M, Cekic O, Yilmaz OF. Combined intravitreal bevacizumab and triamcinolone injection in a child with Coats' disease. J AAPOS. 2008;12(3):309–11.
10. Eagle RC Jr. Eye pathology. Philadelphia: Lippincott & Williams; 2011. p. 221–2.
11. Shields JA, et al. Classification and management of Coats' disease: the 2000 proctor lecture. Am J Ophthalmol. 2001;131(5):572–83.

12. Bindoff LA, et al. Severe facioscapulohumeral muscular dystrophy presenting with Coats' disease and mental retardation. Neuromuscul Disord. 2006;16(9–10):559–63.
13. Beby F, et al. Coats' disease and bilateral cataract in a child with turner syndrome: a case report. Graefes Arch Clin Exp Ophthalmol. 2005;243(12):1291–3.
14. Schuman JS, et al. Senior-Loken syndrome (familial renal-retinal dystrophy) and Coats' disease. Am J Ophthalmol. 1985;100(6):822–7.
15. Mansukhani S, et al. Cerebroretinal microangiopathy with calcifications and cysts (CRMCC) or "Coats' plus": when peripheral retinal vasculature signals neurologic disease. J AAPOS. 2017;21(5):420–2.
16. Kumar V, Chandra P, Kumar A. Ultra-wide field imaging in the diagnosis and management of adult-onset Coats' disease. Clin Exp Optom. 2017;100(1):79–82.
17. Grosso A, et al. Pearls and pitfalls in diagnosis and management of Coats' disease. Retina. 2015;35(4):614–23.
18. Sigler EJ, Calzada JI. Retinal angiomatous proliferation with chorioretinal anastomosis in childhood Coats' disease: a reappraisal of macular fibrosis using multimodal imaging. Retina. 2015;35(3):537–46.
19. Rabiolo A, et al. Refining Coats' disease by ultra-wide-field imaging and optical coherence tomography angiography. Graefes Arch Clin Exp Ophthalmol. 2017;255(10):1881–90.
20. Kumar P, Kumar V. Vitrectomy for epiretinal membrane in adult-onset Coats' disease. Indian J Ophthalmol. 2017;65(10):1046–8.
21. Rishi P, et al. Coats' disease: an Indian perspective. Indian J Ophthalmol. 2010;58(2):119–24.
22. Beselga D, et al. Refractory Coats' disease of adult onset. Case Rep Ophthalmol. 2012;3(1):118–22.
23. Jarin RR, Teoh SC, Lim TH. Resolution of severe macular oedema in adult Coats' syndrome with high-dose intravitreal triamcinolone acetonide. Eye (Lond). 2006;20(2):163–5.
24. London NJS, Shields CL, Haller JA. Chapter 56—Coats disease. In: Ryan SJ, Sadda SVR, Hinton DR, Schachat AP, Sadda SVR, Wilkinson CP, Wiedemann P, Schachat AP, editors. Retina. 5th ed. Philadelphia: W.B. Saunders; 2013. p. 1058–70. ISBN: 9781455707379. https://doi.org/10.1016/B978-1-4557-0737-9.00056-4.
25. Shields JA, Shields CL. Differentiation of Coats' disease and retinoblastoma. J Pediatr Ophthalmol Strabismus. 2001;38(5):262–6. quiz 302–3.
26. Nucci P, et al. Selective photocoagulation in Coats' disease: ten-year follow-up. Eur J Ophthalmol. 2002;12(6):501–5.
27. Shapiro MJ, et al. Effects of green diode laser in the treatment of pediatric Coats' disease. Am J Ophthalmol. 2011;151(4):725–731 e2.
28. Cai X, et al. Treatment of stage 3 Coats' disease by endolaser photocoagulation via a two-port pars plana nonvitrectomy approach. Graefes Arch Clin Exp Ophthalmol. 2015;253(7):999–1004.
29. Suesskind D, et al. Pars plana vitrectomy for treatment of advanced Coats' disease—presentation of a modified surgical technique and long-term follow-up. Graefes Arch Clin Exp Ophthalmol. 2014;252(6):873–9.
30. Othman IS, Moussa M, Bouhaimed M. Management of lipid exudates in Coats' disease by adjuvant intravitreal triamcinolone: effects and complications. Br J Ophthalmol. 2010;94(5):606–10.
31. Sun Y, Jain A, Moshfeghi DM. Elevated vascular endothelial growth factor levels in Coats' disease: rapid response to pegaptanib sodium. Graefes Arch Clin Exp Ophthalmol. 2007;245(9):1387–8.
32. He YG, et al. Elevated vascular endothelial growth factor level in Coats' disease and possible therapeutic role of bevacizumab. Graefes Arch Clin Exp Ophthalmol. 2010;248(10):1519–21.
33. Zheng XX, Jiang YR. The effect of intravitreal bevacizumab injection as the initial treatment for Coats' disease. Graefes Arch Clin Exp Ophthalmol. 2014;252(1):35–42.
34. Villegas VM, et al. Advanced Coats' disease treated with intravitreal bevacizumab combined with laser vascular ablation. Clin Ophthalmol. 2014;8:973–6.

35. Gaillard MC, et al. Ranibizumab in the management of advanced Coats' disease stages 3B and 4: long-term outcomes. Retina. 2014;34(11):2275–81.
36. Yang Q, et al. Successful use of intravitreal ranibizumab injection and combined treatment in the management of Coats' disease. Acta Ophthalmol. 2016;94(4):401–6.
37. Guixeres Esteve MC, Pardo Saiz AO. Coats' disease with macular oedema responsive to aflibercept and argon laser. Arch Soc Esp Oftalmol. 2017;92(7):330–3.
38. Kase S, et al. Expression of vascular endothelial growth factor in eyes with Coats' disease. Invest Ophthalmol Vis Sci. 2013;54(1):57–62.
39. Ramasubramanian A, Shields CL. Bevacizumab for Coats' disease with exudative retinal detachment and risk of vitreoretinal traction. Br J Ophthalmol. 2012;96(3):356–9.
40. Daruich A, et al. Extramacular fibrosis in Coats' disease. Retina. 2016;36(10):2022–8.
41. Sein J, et al. Treatment of Coats' disease with combination therapy of Intravitreal Bevacizumab, laser photocoagulation, and sub-tenon corticosteroids. Ophthalmic Surg Lasers Imaging Retina. 2016;47(5):443–9.
42. Al-Qahtani AA, Almasaud JM, Ghazi NG. Clinical characteristics and treatment outcomes of Coats' disease in a Saudi Arabian population. Retina. 2015;35(10):2091–9.

Management of Choroidal Hemangioma

Brent E. Aebi and Denis Jusufbegovic

Abbreviations

CCH	Circumscribed choroidal hemangioma
CME	Cystoid macular edema
CNV	Choroidal neovascularization
DCH	Diffuse choroidal hemangioma
ERD	Exudative retinal detachment
FA	Fluorescein angiography
ICG-A	Indocyanine green angiography
IVB	Intravitreal bevacizumab
IVT	Intravitreal triamcinolone
LSRT	Lens-sparing radiotherapy
MRI	Magnetic resonance imaging
NVD	Neovascularization of the disc
NVE	Retinal neovascularization elsewhere
OCT	Optical coherence tomography
OCT-A	Optical coherence tomography angiography
PDT	Photodynamic therapy
RPE	Retinal pigment epithelium
SRF	Subretinal fluid
SWS	Sturge-Weber syndrome
TTT	Transpupillary thermotherapy
VEGF	Vascular endothelial growth factor

B. E. Aebi · D. Jusufbegovic (✉)
Department of Ophthalmology, Indiana University School of Medicine,
Eugene and Marilyn Glick Eye Institute, Indianapolis, IN, USA
e-mail: baebi@iu.edu; djusufbe@iu.edu

© Springer Nature Singapore Pte Ltd. 2019
A. Ramasubramanian (ed.), *Ocular Oncology*, Current Practices in
Ophthalmology, https://doi.org/10.1007/978-981-13-7538-5_8

Introduction

Choroidal hemangiomas are relatively rare benign hamartomatous vascular tumors affecting the choroid. They present in two distinct forms, either as a circumscribed or diffuse choroidal lesion. Both forms are thought to be congenital in nature. Circumscribed choroidal hemangioma (CCH) usually presents as a unilateral, solitary choroidal mass with median age at onset in the fourth to fifth decades of life. They have the highest incidence in Caucasian patients and equally affect men and women [1–3].

Diffuse choroidal hemangiomas (DCH) are strongly associated with Sturge-Weber syndrome (SWS). They typically present ipsilateral to the nevus flammeus or port-wine stain, although bilateral cases have been reported. DCH appears as a diffuse, orange thickening of the choroid and has been described as a "tomato catsup" fundus. DCH is highly associated with amblyopia [4, 5].

It is difficult to obtain a precise incidence and prevalence of choroidal hemangiomas in the general population, given their relative rarity as well as the fact that they are only discovered when symptomatic or during routine eye examinations. Two reports from tertiary referral centers estimate the discovery of one circumscribed choroidal hemangioma for every 15–50 newly diagnosed ocular melanomas [6, 7].

Exudative retinal detachment (ERD) is a major clinical feature of both CCH and DCH and is the typical etiology of decreased visual acuity in these patients, which is the most common presenting symptom. ERD occurs secondary to fluid leakage from the hemangioma into the subretinal space and is associated with degenerative changes in the fundus [8].

Clinical Features and Diagnosis

Clinical Presentation

Circumscribed Choroidal Hemangioma

CCH presents as a solitary indistinct pinkish-orange choroidal mass with a median age at onset of symptoms in the fourth to fifth decades of life. Patients most commonly present with decreased vision secondary to serous retinal detachment [1, 2].

In the largest retrospective review of CCH cases, the most frequently reported symptom was decreased visual acuity in 81% of patients. Much less frequently reported symptoms included visual field defects, metamorphopsia, and floaters. The vast majority of patients were Caucasian (92%) with a mean age of onset of 45 years (range 4–77 years). Twenty-four percent of patients presented with acuity of 20/40 or better while 53% of patients presented with acuity of 20/200 or worse; of note 10% of patients included in the above observational study had received prior treatment. CCH was associated with subretinal fluid at the site of the tumor in 81% of cases. Retinal pigment epithelial (RPE) hyperplasia was present overlying 33% of CCH with RPE metaplasia present in 20%. The mean tumor diameter was 6.7 mm (range 3–16 mm) with a mean tumor thickness as measured by ultrasound of 3.1 mm (range 1–8 mm). Two-thirds of CCH were located in the macula with one-third located outside the macula but posterior to the equator [3].

There are rare reports of choroidal neovascularization (CNV) in treatment-naïve eyes with CCH [9, 10]. While DCH is highly associated with SWS, there are rare case reports of CCH occurring in patients with SWS, with or without concurrent DCH [5, 11].

Diffuse Choroidal Hemangioma

DCH presents as a diffuse orange thickening of the choroid and is highly associated with Sturge-Weber syndrome. The lesion is typically unilateral and ipsilateral to the nevus flammeus. DCH can be associated with sectoral iris hemangioma or iris mammillations, which can present as iris heterochromia [12, 13]. Patients with DCH have a high incidence of amblyopia.

Clinical Course

In a review of 82 patients with CCH presenting with poor visual acuity defined as 20/200 or worse, 54% had poor visual acuity at 5-year and 80% at 10-year follow-up. Predictors of poor visual outcome include poor initial visual acuity, failure of previous laser photocoagulation, and tumor management with observation [3, 14]. Over time, CCH may undergo very gradual but progressive enlargement [15].

As DCH commonly causes poor vision in infants, it is highly associated with amblyopia even after treatment and subsequent resolution of a retinal detachment and frequently is associated with poor visual outcomes. A review of 33 SWS patients showed that 67% of eyes with DCH had severely impaired long-term vision [4]. Of note, patients with SWS can also have vision abnormalities secondary to leptomeningeal angioma or glaucoma [16].

Clinical Features

Fundus Examination—As many choroidal hemangiomas are diagnosed after the onset of secondary ERD, the main clinical finding is significant areas of subretinal fluid (SRF) with retinal elevation. CCH typically presents as a subtle pinkish-orange mass with indistinct margins identified in the macula in 67% of patients (Fig. 1a), while tumors in the nasal and superior periphery have been reported in 14% and 11% of patients, respectively. DCH in the setting of SWS presents with the typical tomato-catsup fundus and thickening of the posterior choroid (Fig. 2a) [3, 17].

Fluorescein Angiography (FA)—FA is a helpful ancillary test in evaluating CCH and typically shows a lacy hyperfluorescence in the early arterial phase characteristic of highly vascular lesions (Fig. 1b). There is usually persistent hyperfluorescence of the lesion throughout the angiographic study with late staining in a multiloculated pattern and a variable amount of fluorescein leakage (Fig. 3a). At times, a hypofluorescent zone at the tumor margin suggests blockage by melanocytes. Despite its usefulness, FA patterns in CCH may be variable and can simulate other choroidal lesions. Thus, the importance of ophthalmoscopic appearance and other ancillary test findings in ruling out similar lesions cannot be overstated.

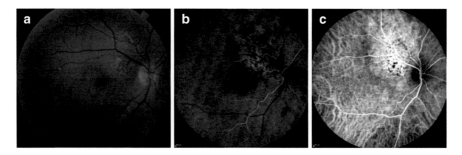

Fig. 1 (a) Color fundus photograph demonstrates pinkish-orange choroidal mass with indistinct borders. Overlying orange (lipofuscin) pigment is also present, which can be seen in different amounts in up to one-third of active lesions. (b) Early arterial phase of fluorescein angiogram shows lacy, patchy hyperfluorescence of the lesion. (c) Maximal hyperfluorescence with hypofluorescent spots is seen in the venous phase of indocyanine green angiogram

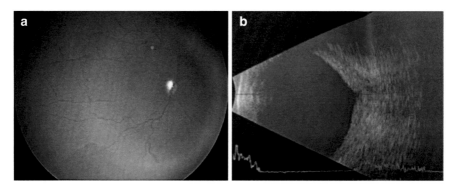

Fig. 2 (a) Deep red-pink appearance of the fundus (tomato-catsup fundus) is seen in this case of diffuse choroidal hemangioma. Cupping of the optic nerve is also present, which is a common complication of Sturge-Weber syndrome. (b) B-scan ultrasound demonstrates diffuse thickening of the choroid

Leakage is not a feature readily encountered in DCH, although it aids in visualization of SRF when present [18, 19].

Indocyanine Green Angiography (ICG-A)—ICG-A provides an excellent view of choroidal tumors given its propensity in evaluating choroidal vasculature. Hyperfluorescence of tumor vessels against a hypofluorescent background is present in the arterial phase. Hyper- and hypofluorescent spots are seen at the stage of maximal fluorescence in the venous phase (Fig. 1c). In CCH, late frames commonly exhibit hyperfluorescence of the tumor margin and scattered hot spots. Later frames show a characteristic decrease in fluorescence and commonly demonstrate "washout" appearance of the lesion (Fig. 3b). In patients with DCH, areas outside the tumor can exhibit hyperfluorescence as well [17, 20].

Ultrasonography—CCH: A-scan shows a high peak at the anterior surface of tumor with increased internal reflectivity between 50 and 100% differentiating CCH

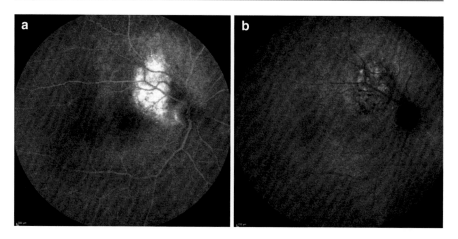

Fig. 3 (**a**) Persistent hyperfluorescence with staining and small amount of leakage is present in very late stages of the fluorescein angiogram, as opposed to (**b**) characteristic hypofluorescence, also known as "washout" appearance, that can be appreciated in the late frames of indocyanine green angiogram

from the lower internal reflectivity present in ocular melanoma. B-scan shows an elevated acoustically solid mass [17, 21].

DCH: Choroidal mass is visible on B-scan with diffuse thickening of the choroid and medium-to-high internal reflectivity (Fig. 2b) [22, 23].

Optical Coherence Tomography (OCT)—OCT with enhanced depth imaging is useful in the evaluation of CCH and DCH. OCT is able to readily delineate choroidal tumors from surrounding healthy tissue aiding in the measurement of tumors. The tumor demonstrates a medium-to-low reflective band with posterior shadowing. OCT angiography (OCT-A) has demonstrated large choroidal vessels inside CCH and an irregular dense vascular network in the deep outer retinal layer. Even without OCT-A, expansion of choroidal vessels is apparent on OCT [24–26].

Magnetic Resonance Imaging (MRI)—MRI has been employed to guide the differential diagnosis of CH. The most useful series in the differentiation between CCH and choroidal melanoma tends to be the T2 series, which shows CCH isointense to the vitreous in more than 93% of cases. Melanoma is hypointense on T2 in 93–95% of cases. Metastatic lesions also tend to be isointense on T2. Post-contrast images show a greater increase in signal for CCH versus melanoma. T1 images are less helpful in the differentiation of choroidal tumors. While T2 FLAIR demonstrates high-quality resolution of tumors, both melanoma and choroidal hemangiomas are hyperintense in this series [27–29]. Compared to the vitreous, DCH is hyperintense on the T1 series and isointense on T2 [22].

Fundus Autofluorescence (FAF)—Areas with orange pigment overlying CCH demonstrate hyperautofluorescence as well as fresh SRF. RPE hyperplasia, fibrous metaplasia, and atrophy, which can all be associated with CCH, show hypoautofluo-rescence. DCH is hypoautofluorescent but after treatment can show hyperautofluo-rescence [30].

Differential Diagnoses
- Amelanotic choroidal melanoma
- Choroidal metastasis
- Choroidal osteoma
- Inflammatory processes
- Dome-shaped macula
- Choroidal nevus
- Choroidal granuloma
- Age-related macular degeneration
- Central serous chorioretinopathy
- Retinoblastoma

Management of Choroidal Hemangioma

Laser and Phototherapy

Laser Photocoagulation
Xenon and argon lasers have been an effective treatment for both CCH for many years with resolution of subretinal fluid in the majority of patients and stabilization of vision in 53–71% of patients. Some patients demonstrate temporary improve-ment of vision with long-term worsening. One case series noted a 40% fluid recur-rence rate after treatment of CCH [3, 31].

However, with the advent of phototherapy, photocoagulation is now rarely per-formed in the treatment of CCH as photocoagulation cannot be used to treat subfo-veal tumors and results in large areas of RPE atrophy [32].

Transpupillary Thermotherapy
Transpupillary thermotherapy (TTT) can be used to treat extrafoveal, post-equatorial CCH with small amounts of SRF. The ideal tumor for treatment with TTT is less than 10 mm in diameter and less than 4 mm thick. TTT increases the internal tem-perature of a tumor to 40 °C (65 °C at the tumor apex) causing a cytotoxic effect and sclerosis of vascular tumors. TTT utilizes an 810 nm diode laser with a large spot size and long exposure time. Risks of TTT include cystoid macular edema (CME), preretinal fibrosis, iris atrophy, retinal vascular occlusion, and thermal papillitis if treating a tumor in contact with the optic disc [33, 34].

In a summary of six combined case series, visual acuity improved in 40–75% of patients and tumor size decreased in most patients [34, 35]. Approximately 42% of tumors showed complete regression while 53% underwent partial regression. There was greater improvement when treated within 6 months of the onset of symptoms [3, 34].

Given the focal nature of TTT, it does not lend itself to treating DCH. However, treatment of DCH with TTT has been reported to lower intraocular pressure in two patients with SWS and juvenile-onset glaucoma. Neither patient had ERD at the time of treatment [36].

Photodynamic Therapy (PDT)

Photodynamic therapy (PDT) is the most widely used treatment in choroidal hemangioma and has become the treatment of choice, especially for subfoveal CCH. As a selective vaso-occlusive treatment, PDT was first used to target tumor vasculature by oncologists. The first ophthalmic use of PDT was the treatment of CNV in the foveal region associated with age-related macular degeneration in the 1990s. PDT utilizes a photosensitizing agent that undergoes a photochemical reaction when activated, producing secondary occlusion of vasculature limited to the treatment area of the light source. Verteporfin is the photosensitizing agent of choice given its lipophilicity, its short half-life in serum, and its absorption spectrum. While its absorption spectrum is broad, typically 689 nm, in the far-red region, it is used clinically. Melanin, blood, and fibrous tissue are easily penetrable at this wavelength, making it ideal for treatment of the choroid. Verteporfin is sequestered in vessels with a larger caliber and has minimal accumulation in the healthy capillaries of the choroid [33, 37, 38].

Three variables contribute to the precise treatment of a choroidal vascular lesion:

- Verteporfin dose
- Duration of verteporfin infusion
- Light dose [37]

Standard dosing of verteporfin consists of 6 mg/m^2 of body surface area, infused over a 10-min period with treatment typically at 15 min. A 50 J/cm^2 concentration of light energy is achieved by using a light source of 600 mW/cm^2 with 83 s of exposure. Standard dosing has been shown to be both safe and effective. By doubling the time of exposure to 166 s, exposure with 100 J/cm^2 is achieved. PDT typically reduces tumor thickness, but resolution of SRF is considered the endpoint of therapy and it has shown promising results in the correction of ERD. Often, only one treatment is required; occasionally two or even three treatments are required [37, 39, 40]. PDT can be given as a single-spot or with overlapping spot therapy. A small study was unable to demonstrate a significant difference in visual outcomes, but either of these two strategies can be employed, especially as tumor size is considered [41]. PDT has an excellent safety profile [42].

While standard dosing with verteporfin involves slow infusion of 6 mg/m^2 over 10 min, injecting this same dose as a bolus over 1 min has been shown to be noninferior. However, it is postulated that this may be more likely to lead to changes in both the retina and RPE and might result in reduced retinal sensitivity [40]. Treatment of a single patient with a half-dose bolus of 3 mg/m^2 over 1 min was shown to be effective in treating a small ERD with improvement of visual acuity from 20/30 to 20/20 [43].

PDT for Circumscribed Choroidal Hemangioma

As the most popular treatment for CCH, there are many case series—both prospective and retrospective—as well as reviews of PDT in the literature which describe good outcomes for patients treated with PDT [39, 44–48]. No randomized controlled trials have been conducted to date. While not an exhaustive list, several larger case series are described in Table 1.

Table 1 PDT for circumscribed choroidal hemangioma

Study	Treatment	Follow-up period [36]	Findings
Boixadera et al. (2009) – 31 patients – Prospective – Multicenter trial [82]	Standard protocol	12 months	– 17.2% of patients required more than one treatment session – 69% of patients with visual recovery – SRF resolved in all but 2 cases – Mean visual acuity increased from 20/60 to 20/35 – CCH thickness decreased in all cases (mean 3.0–1.7 mm) – Peak tumor regression 4 weeks after therapy – No severe adverse events
Jurklies et al. (2003) – 19 patients – Prospective – Case series [83]	100 J/cm^2, *otherwise settings consistent with standard protocol*	10.6-month mean follow-up {2–24}	– Visual acuity improved in 73.3% patients – Acuity improved ≥2 lines in 42.1% – Regression of tumor height in all 19 tumors – Risk factors for no improvement: – Symptoms >30 months – Decreased acuity – Any pretreatment (irradiation or photocoagulation) – No significant response after first PDT session
Michels et al. (2005) – 15 patients – Prospective – Case series [84]	100 J/cm^2, *otherwise settings consistent with standard protocol*	36.6-month mean follow-up {12–50}	– All patients: – Complete regression of tumor – No tumor growth on follow-up – No SRF recurrence – 13 patients gained 2–9 lines of acuity
Schmidt-Erfurth et al. (2002) – 15 patients – Prospective – Case series [38]	100 J/cm^2, *otherwise settings consistent with standard protocol*	19-month mean follow-up {12–50}	– Complete regression of mass – Most intensive effect after first application – 13 patients with visual recovery – 2 patients with stable visual acuity and resolution of metamorphopsia – Mean acuity improved from 20/125 to 20/80

Table 1 (continued)

Study	Treatment	Follow-up period [36]	Findings
Verbraak et al. (2003) – 13 patients – Case series – Consecutive patients [85]	10 patients. -> Standard protocol 3 patients. -> 100 J/cm², *otherwise settings consistent with standard protocol*	12-month mean follow-up {3–22}	– 2 patients previously treated with radiation – Visual acuity improved in 11 non-previously treated patients – 9 patients with undetectable tumor by ultrasound 6 weeks after treatment – 4 patients with undetectable tumor after second PDT session – No increase in acuity for 2 patients previously treated with radiation; they did report widened visual field and sharper vision – Low energy 50 J/cm² did not appear to be inferior to 100 J/cm²
Singh et al. (2004) – 10 patients – Prospective – Consecutive patients – Case series [86]	Standard protocol	7-month median follow-up {1–13}	– 2 cases previously treated with TTT – 1 case s/p external beam radiotherapy – All patients: – Flattening of tumor – SRF resolution – Reduced choroidal vasculature on angiogram – Acuity improved or remained stable in 80% – 2 patients with vision loss secondary to delayed choroidal atrophy
Porrini et al. (2003) – 10 patients – Prospective – Consecutive patients – Case series [87]	*Lesions >2 mm* 100 J/cm² *Lesions <2 mm* 75 J/cm², *otherwise settings consistent with standard protocol*	{7–16 months}	– Visual acuity improved in all cases – 4 cases improved to 20/20 (3 tumors extrafoveal; 1 subfoveal) – 4 cases required 3 PDT treatments – ERD resolved in all cases – 6 cases with no measurable tumor height by ultrasound after treatment – Alterations in RPE noted for 50% of patients with 3 PDT treatment sessions – No RPE changes observed in patients after 2 PDT sessions

*Standard protocol =
– Verteporfin dosing: 6 mg/m² of body surface area infused over 10 min
– Laser settings: 50 J/cm², 600 mW/cm², duration 83 s (689–692 nm)

PDT for Diffuse Choroidal Hemangioma

In patients with DCH, PDT has been shown to cause tumor regression and treat associated ERD. A case series of six patients with DCH, three of whom presented with secondary ERD, had the following findings:

– All six tumors regressed
– Two of three ERD resolved completely

- Two patients required more than one treatment session
- Acuity improved in three cases, but was limited by amblyopia in three cases [49]

The youngest case report for successful PDT treatment of ERD in the setting of SWS involved a 6-year-old with DCH. She had a history of no light perception vision in her fellow eye with unsuccessful PDT at age 3. At age 6 she developed progressive blurring of vision to 20/50. She was treated with standard protocol PDT guided by fluorescein angiography and experienced resolution of SRF and maintenance of 20/50 vision [50].

There are several other case reports in the literature that show complete SRF resolution and improvement in visual acuity after a single PDT treatment in patients with SWS and DCH using the above standard protocol [19, 32, 51, 52].

PDT has been demonstrated to decrease choroidal thickness by about 65% in a single patient from 251 to 83 μm [53]. However this measurement is somewhat limited given the normal diurnal variation in choroidal thickness, which can vary up to 43.1 μm in a healthy choroid. It is also difficult to measure the thickness throughout the entire choroid as opposed to the subfoveal measurement alone [54].

Complications

While CNV is a rare finding in treatment-naïve eyes with CCH, PDT has been shown to worsen preexisting CNV [9]. PDT might also cause CNV [55]. In three eyes with neovascularization of the disc (NVD) or neovascularization elsewhere (NVE) prior to PDT, neovascularization worsened after treatment. These patients were successfully treated with intravitreal triamcinolone (IVT) [9].

Pharmacologic Therapy

Anti-VEGF therapy

Another relatively new trend to emerge in the treatment of choroidal hemangiomas is the use of intravitreal agents targeted against vascular endothelial growth factor (VEGF). These medications have been shown to be useful therapy in the treatment of choroidal hemangiomas, either as solo therapy or in conjunction with other treatment modalities. Intravitreal anti-VEGF can be used to augment therapy with PDT, photocoagulation, or TTT and many vitreoretinal specialists use a combined approach when treating DCH or CCH [7, 10, 56, 57, 58, 59].

Anti-VEGF acts directly against the vasculature of the tumor and can cause a decrease in size of the tumor as well as reduction or even complete resolution of ERD. Intravitreal bevacizumab (IVB) is the most commonly reported medication in the literature given its availability and relatively low cost compared with other anti-VEGF agents. Intravitreal bevacizumab, ranibizumab, aflibercept, and even pegaptanib have all been used to treat both CCH and DCH with no evidence to suggest the superiority or inferiority of any particular agent; no study approaching a comparative trial has been performed to date [10, 44, 60].

Anti-VEGF Therapy for Circumscribed Choroidal Hemangioma

Recently, the practice of pretreating ERD with intravitreal anti-VEGF medication followed by PDT has increased. Results have been promising thus far with complete resolution of SRF and either improvement or stabilization of visual acuity with a stable exam over time and no recurrence of fluid after therapy [7, 57, 59].

Three cases have been reported with IVB used for ERD refractory to treatment with laser photocoagulation. ERD resolved in all three patients after undergoing IVB treatment. Stable chronic cystoid macular changes remained in two patients, but they had no recurrence of retinal detachment [56, 57].

Anti-VEGF therapy has been used to treat CNV occurring along with CCH or as a result of photodynamic therapy with good results [10, 60].

Anti-VEGF Therapy for Diffuse Choroidal Hemangioma

Intravitreal anti-VEGF has been used as solo therapy to treat the ERD associated with DCH in patients with SWS. The number of monthly treatments required for complete resolution of the retinal detachment varies, but multiple cases have completely resolved after a single treatment with intravitreal bevacizumab without recurrence of SRF [7, 61, 62].

Treatment of an ERD secondary to DCH with PDT followed by intravitreal injection of bevacizumab several days later has been shown to completely resolve ERD associated with no recurrence of fluid at 18 months with preserved visual acuity [58].

Beta-Blockers

Nonselective beta-blockers have been used for various capillary hemangiomas, both topically and systemically. Oral propranolol has been beneficial in treating choroidal hemangiomas. The effect of propranolol is thought to occur by acting on capillaries by three mechanisms:

1. Vasoconstriction
2. Downregulation of the RAF-mitogen-activated protein kinase pathway resulting in downstream decreased expression of VEGF, beta-fibroblast growth factor (βFGF), and hypoxia-inducible factor 1 alpha (HIF-1α)
3. Inducing apoptosis of endothelial cells [8, 63, 64]

Propranolol for Circumscribed Choroidal Hemangioma

Beta-blockers are often not effective in completely resolving SRF associated with CCH. Six published cases of CCH in adults treated with oral propranolol are summarized in Table 2. Propranolol has been shown to decrease, and at times completely resolve, SRF associated with ERD. It does not appear to have any effect on

Table 2   Treatment of circumscribed choroidal hemangioma with oral propranolol

Age/gender	Maximum dose used	Change in SRF
51 male [14]	50 mg TID	Decrease in focal areas of SRF, increase in CME over time
44 female [14]	30 mg TID	Decrease in SRF
59 male [14]	20 mg TID	Complete resolution of ERD
42 male [14]	40 mg TID	No SRF on presentation
41 female [14]	30 mg TID	Decrease in SRF
59 male [65]	120 mg daily	Complete resolution of ERD

No patients experienced decrease in size of CCH

Table 3   Treatment of diffuse choroidal hemangioma with oral propranolol

Age/gender	Maximum dose used	Change in SRF	Acuity
14 male [88]	1 mg/kg/day	Complete resolution of ERD with 8 weeks of treatment	CF at 3 m improved to 20/30
58 female [23]	80 mg BID	Complete resolution of ERD with 6 weeks of treatment	LP vision improved to HM
5 male [89]	40 mg BID, slowly weaned to 10 mg	ERD receded to peripheral retina after 6 months	*None reported*
17 male [67]	60 mg BID	Complete resolution of ERD with 1 month of treatment Decrease in size of DCH	20/60 vision remained stable
14 female [22]	2 mg/kg/day	Complete resolution of ERD with 6 months of therapy	History of poor vision OS (HM) since birth, no final acuity reported
59 male [22]	2 mg/kg/day	No SRF on presentation No occurrence of SRF No decrease in size of tumor	NLP OD, 20/300 OS with no change in acuity Patient with history of bilateral glaucoma requiring tube shunts

decreasing the overall size of the tumor. One patient had an increase in CME over time as focal areas of SRF resolved. Given these reported cases, a 120 mg daily dose appears to be both safe and effective if beta-blockade will help resolve ERD in any given patient. If a patient does not respond to this dose, it is reasonable to abandon treatment with propranolol and consider other therapy for SRF [14, 65].

Propranolol for Diffuse Choroidal Hemangioma

While the results of beta-blockers in the treatment of CCH have been mixed, oral propranolol has shown much more promise in the treatment of DCH in reported cases. There are five reported cases of ERD secondary to DCH treated with oral propranolol. A sixth patient was treated prophylactically to prevent occurrence of SRF [22]. These results are summarized in Table 3. SRF completely resolved in 80% of patients treated over a relatively short period of time, including one individual with an ERD for 3 years prior to initiating treatment [66]. The size of choroidal hemangioma decreased in one individual [67]. Amblyopia as well as other visual comorbidities played a role in these patients with DCH in the setting of SWS.

Intravitreal Triamcinolone

With the increased use of anti-VEGF therapy in recent years, intravitreal steroids have decreased in their frequency of use, presumably given the difference in long-term risk for complications, including increased risk for glaucoma. However, IVT remains an option in the treatment of choroidal hemangioma and its sequelae. IVT has been used for two indications associated with CCH.

The first indication was demonstrated in a case series; IVT was used in conjunction with PDT to treat ERD in four eyes. Three eyes obtained resolution of SRF, but one eye had persistent ERD. All ten eyes treated with PDT alone achieved complete resolution of SRF. It is noted in patients treated with IVT in addition to PDT; 2/4 patients had improvement of visual acuity greater than two lines, whereas only 3/10 eyes had visual acuity improvement greater than two lines when treated with PDT alone. The other seven eyes had acuity which remained stable. Given the low sample size and lack of control for other factors that could influence visual outcome, it is difficult to confirm benefit from the addition of IVT to PDT [45].

The second indication for IVT is for a very few reported cases of neovascularization associated with CCH. As mentioned above, the occurrence of neovascularization in the setting of CCH is rare, but when present PDT has been shown to worsen the amount of NVD or NVE. IVT has been used to effectively resolve both worsened NVD and NVE after PDT [9].

Intravitreal Dexamethasone Implant

A single case is reported in which intravitreal dexamethasone implant was used prior to PDT therapy to treat ERD with secondary resolution of SRF and flattening of the primary CCH [68]. Intravitreal dexamethasone has also been used to treat recurrent SRF after undergoing PDT in a few cases [44, 69].

Radiation Therapy

Plaque Brachytherapy

Episcleral brachytherapy involves placing radioactive plaques external to a choroidal tumor and has been used to treat CCH. A variety of isotopes have been employed including cobalt-60, iodine-125, ruthenium-106, and palladium-103 over several case series, with similar results. Treatment in four case series showed a mean reduction in tumor height ranging from 44 to 57% and vision stabilized in ≥75% or more of patients, when reported. Brachytherapy does require a patient to undergo two surgeries—one to place the radioactive material and the other for removal [70–73].

A retrospective case series details ruthenium-106 plaque therapy in five eyes with DCH:

- All five eyes had complete tumor regression.
- Both eyes with SRF prior to treatment had complete resolution of fluid.
- One eye with secondary glaucoma progressed to NLP.
- Two eyes had improvement in visual acuity.
- No radiation-induced complications were observed in any patients [74].

Proton Therapy

Proton beam radiotherapy is one of the leading treatments for uveal melanoma and a low-dose proton therapy has also been used in the treatment of CCH. Two large case series (summarized in Table 4) used a 20 cobalt gray equivalent dose of radiation given over 4 days after suturing tantalum clips to the sclera to delineate the margins of the hemangioma. Retinal reattachment occurred in all cases with resolution of ERD. Radiation can be delivered as a homogenous dose and spares healthy retinal tissue surrounding the tumor [75, 76].

In six DCH treated with proton beam irradiation, three eyes had improvement of visual acuity. When assessing tumor regression, visual acuity, and resolution of SRF outcomes were similar between DCH and CCH, although on average there was increased time to fluid resolution in DCH compared with CCH. The rate of radiation complications was comparable between the two types of tumor [77].

Proton beam therapy exposes the anterior eye to higher levels of radiation than brachytherapy. Proton therapy also requires a single surgical procedure to place the tantalum clips as opposed to two procedures required for brachytherapy. Late complications of therapy include radiation maculopathy, optic neuropathy, and cataract formation. An 8% incidence of radiation maculopathy was reported in one study. A macular shield can be used to decrease the radiation dose to the macula by 50% [75, 76]. In general, the incidence of radiation retinopathy is low following a low-dose proton therapy.

Table 4 Low-dose proton therapy for circumscribed choroidal hemangioma

Levy-Gabriel et al. [76]	Frau et al. [75]
- Retrospective case series	- Retrospective case series
- 71 eyes with CCH	- 17 eyes with CCH
- All tumors decreased in thickness	- All tumors regressed
- 92.5% of eyes developed completely flat scar	- One eye had onset of ERD 1 year after initial treatment -> resolved with second treatment
- Visual acuity improved in 52% of patients	
- Acuity improved in 75% of eyes when treatment initiated within 6 months of symptom onset	- Acuity improved in 94% of eyes and was stable in the remaining eye

External Beam Radiotherapy

Lens-sparing radiotherapy (LSRT) uses a vacuum contact lens and collimators to focus a beam of radiation precisely on a hemangioma and avoid exposing the lens to high doses of radiation, thus delaying the onset of visually significant cataract [78]. Retrospective studies have mixed results. In the largest retrospective paper of 36 CCH and 15 DCH treated with 20 Gy LSRT, results were similar between the two groups. After treatment of patients with CCH, 36.2% had residual ERD, 38.9% had improvement in visual acuity, 38.9% had stable visual acuity, and visual acuity decreased in 22.2%. Visual acuity improved in 46.6% of patients with DCH [78]. In a smaller case series using 20–24 Gy to treat CCH, visual acuity improved in 8/10 eyes, ERD completely resolved in all cases, and tumor regressed in all cases [79].

A small retrospective review comparing photocoagulation, brachytherapy, and LSRT (18–30 Gy) suggested that LSRT was inferior; however it was unevenly skewed as the CCH treated with LSRT was thicker and closer to the fovea. The same study describing five DCH treated with LSRT showed complete resolution of SRF in all cases, stable acuity in three patients, and marked visual improvement in two patients [72].

Gamma Knife

Very few retrospective case series have explored gamma knife radiosurgery for DCH and CCH. One case series used a 10 Gy marginal dose to treat seven eyes with either DCH or CCH. All patients had improvement in visual acuity and complete SRF resolution without recurrence. No radiation toxicity was observed [80]. Gamma knife has also been used as a secondary treatment when the primary treatment modality failed [81].

Practical Pearls and Pitfalls
- Diagnosis of CCH is based on very characteristic ophthalmoscopic and ancillary test findings. However, other choroidal lesions, including metastases and choroidal melanoma, may occasionally simulate CCH. Therefore, evaluation of amelanotic choroidal lesions requires a careful and methodological approach to minimize a risk of misdiagnosis. Unusual clinical behavior should prompt a clinician to reconsider the established diagnosis.
- PDT with or without anti-VEGF injections has become the treatment of choice for patients with symptomatic CCH with SRF. Radiotherapy is usually an effective alternative for lesions that are nonresponsive or not amenable to laser therapies (PDT, photocoagulation, or TTT). Pharmacotherapies are emerging as a viable option in selected cases; however, more robust clinical trials are required to demonstrate their efficacy. Regardless of treatment modality, delaying therapy tends to result in lower overall visual prognosis when SRF is present.

– DCH is almost universally associated with Sturge-Weber syndrome and presents with diffuse thickening of choroid ipsilateral to facial nevus flammeus. Oral propranolol is more effective in DCH than in CCH; however, other treatment modalities including radiotherapy might be necessary to control chronic exudation.

References

1. Witschel H, Font RL. Hemangioma of the choroid. A clinicopathologic study of 71 cases and a review of the literature. Surv Ophthalmol. 1976;20(6):415–31.
2. Mashayekhi A, Shields CL. Circumscribed choroidal hemangioma. Curr Opin Ophthalmol. 2003;14(3):142–9.
3. Shields CL, Honavar SG, Shields JA, Cater J, Demirci H. Circumscribed choroidal hemangioma: clinical manifestations and factors predictive of visual outcome in 200 consecutive cases. Ophthalmology. 2001;108(12):2237–48.
4. Koenraads Y, van Egmond-Ebbeling MB, de Boer JH, Imhof SM, Braun KP, Porro GL. Visual outcome in Sturge-Weber syndrome: a systematic review and Dutch multicentre cohort. Acta Ophthalmol. 2016;94(7):638–45. https://doi.org/10.1111/aos.13074.
5. Cheung D, Grey R, Rennie I. Circumscribed choroidal haemangioma in a patient with Sturge Weber syndrome. Eye (Lond). 2000;14(Pt 2):238–40. https://doi.org/10.1038/eye.2000.61.
6. Jarrett WH 2nd, Hagler WS, Larose JH, Shields JA. Clinical experience with presumed hemangioma of the choroid: radioactive phosphorus uptake studies as an aid in differential diagnosis. Trans Sect Ophthalmol Am Acad Ophthalmol Otolaryngol. 1976;81(5):862–70.
7. Hsu CC, Yang CS, Peng CH, Lee FL, Lee SM. Combination photodynamic therapy and intravitreal bevacizumab used to treat circumscribed choroidal hemangioma. J Chin Med Assoc. 2011;74(10):473–7. https://doi.org/10.1016/j.jcma.2011.08.020.
8. Shields JA, Shields CL. Intraocular tumors: an atlas and textbook. 2nd ed. Baltimore: Lippincott Williams & Wilkins; 2008.
9. Leys AM, Silva R, Inhoffen W, Tatar O. Neovascular growth following photodynamic therapy for choroidal hemangioma and neovascular regression after intravitreous injection of triamcinolone. Retina. 2006;26(6):693–7. https://doi.org/10.1097/01.iae.0000236482.40056.fe.
10. Hua R, Zhao N, Hu Y, Zhang CM, Chen L. Circumscribed choroidal hemangioma associated with choroidal neovascularization in a HIV-infected case: photodynamic therapy and intravitreous ranibizumab. Photodiagn Photodyn Ther. 2014;11(3):441–3. https://doi.org/10.1016/j.pdpdt.2014.04.005.
11. Scott IU, Alexandrakis G, Cordahi GJ, Murray TG. Diffuse and circumscribed choroidal hemangiomas in a patient with Sturge-Weber syndrome. Arch Ophthalmol. 1999;117(3):406–7.
12. Shields CL, Atalay HT, Wuthisiri W, Levin AV, Lally SE, Shields JA. Sector iris hemangioma in association with diffuse choroidal hemangioma. J AAPOS. 2015;19(1):83–6. https://doi.org/10.1016/j.jaapos.2014.09.012.
13. Plateroti AM, Plateroti R, Mollo R, Librando A, Contestabile MT, Fenicia V. Sturge-weber syndrome associated with monolateral ocular melanocytosis, Iris mammillations, and diffuse choroidal haemangioma. Case Rep Ophthalmol. 2017;8(2):375–84. https://doi.org/10.1159/000477612.
14. Tanabe H, Sahashi K, Kitano T, Tomita Y, Saito AM, Hirose H. Effects of oral propranolol on circumscribed choroidal hemangioma: a pilot study. JAMA Ophthalmol. 2013;131(12):1617–22. https://doi.org/10.1001/jamaophthalmol.2013.5669.
15. Medlock RD, Augsburger JJ, Wilkinson CP, Cox MS Jr, Gamel JW, Nicholl J. Enlargement of circumscribed choroidal hemangiomas. Retina. 1991;11(4):385–8.
16. Kwon HJ, Kim M, Lee CS, Lee SC. Treatment of serous macular detachment associated with circumscribed choroidal hemangioma. Am J Ophthalmol. 2012;154(1):137–145.e131. https://doi.org/10.1016/j.ajo.2012.01.007.

17. Schalenbourg A, Piguet B, Zografos L. Indocyanine green angiographic findings in choroidal hemangiomas: a study of 75 cases. Ophthalmologica. 2000;214(4):246–52. https://doi.org/10.1159/000027499.

18. Norton EW, Gutman F. Fluorescein angiography and hemangiomas of the choroid. Arch Ophthalmol. 1967;78(2):121–5.

19. Anand R. Photodynamic therapy for diffuse choroidal hemangioma associated with Sturge Weber syndrome. Am J Ophthalmol. 2003;136(4):758–60.

20. Arevalo JF, Shields CL, Shields JA, Hykin PG, De Potter P. Circumscribed choroidal hemangioma: characteristic features with indocyanine green videoangiography. Ophthalmology. 2000;107(2):344–50.

21. Singh AD, Kaiser PK, Sears JE. Choroidal hemangioma. Ophthalmol Clin N Am. 2005;18(1):151–161, ix. https://doi.org/10.1016/j.ohc.2004.07.004.

22. Krema H, Yousef YA, Durairaj P, Santiago R. Failure of systemic propranolol therapy for choroidal hemangioma of Sturge-Weber syndrome: a report of 2 cases. JAMA Ophthalmol. 2013;131(5):681–3. https://doi.org/10.1001/jamaophthalmol.2013.2879.

23. Arevalo JF, Arias JD, Serrano MA. Oral propranolol for exudative retinal detachment in diffuse choroidal hemangioma. Arch Ophthalmol. 2011;129(10):1373–5. https://doi.org/10.1001/archophthalmol.2011.294.

24. Cennamo G, Romano MR, Breve MA, Velotti N, Reibaldi M, de Crecchio G, Cennamo G. Evaluation of choroidal tumors with optical coherence tomography: enhanced depth imaging and OCT-angiography features. Eye (Lond). 2017;31(6):906–15. https://doi.org/10.1038/eye.2017.14.

25. Torres VL, Brugnoni N, Kaiser PK, Singh AD. Optical coherence tomography enhanced depth imaging of choroidal tumors. Am J Ophthalmol. 2011;151(4):586–593.e582. https://doi.org/10.1016/j.ajo.2010.09.028.

26. Shields CL, Manalac J, Das C, Saktanasate J, Shields JA. Review of spectral domain enhanced depth imaging optical coherence tomography of tumors of the choroid. Indian J Ophthalmol. 2015;63(2):117–21. https://doi.org/10.4103/0301-4738.154377.

27. Stroszczynski C, Hosten N, Bornfeld N, Wiegel T, Schueler A, Foerster P, Lemke AJ, Hoffmann KT, Felix R. Choroidal hemangioma: MR findings and differentiation from uveal melanoma. Am J Neuroradiol. 1998;19(8):1441–7.

28. Peyster RG, Augsburger JJ, Shields JA, Hershey BL, Eagle R Jr, Haskin ME. Intraocular tumors: evaluation with MR imaging. Radiology. 1988;168(3):773–9. https://doi.org/10.1148/radiology.168.3.3406407.

29. Damento GM, Koeller KK, Salomao DR, Pulido JS. T2 fluid-attenuated inversion recovery imaging of uveal melanomas and other ocular pathology. Ocular Oncol Pathol. 2016;2(4):251–61. https://doi.org/10.1159/000447265.

30. Ramasubramanian A, Shields CL, Harmon SA, Shields JA. Autofluorescence of choroidal hemangioma in 34 consecutive eyes. Retina. 2010;30(1):16–22. https://doi.org/10.1097/IAE.0b013e3181bceedb.

31. Anand R, Augsburger JJ, Shields JA. Circumscribed choroidal hemangiomas. Arch Ophthalmol. 1989;107(9):1338–42.

32. Tsipursky MS, Golchet PR, Jampol LM. Photodynamic therapy of choroidal hemangioma in Sturge-Weber syndrome, with a review of treatments for diffuse and circumscribed choroidal hemangiomas. Surv Ophthalmol. 2011;56(1):68–85. https://doi.org/10.1016/j.survophthal.2010.08.002.

33. Karimi S, Nourinia R, Mashayekhi A. Circumscribed choroidal hemangioma. J Ophthalmic Vis Res. 2015;10(3):320–8. https://doi.org/10.4103/2008-322x.170353.

34. Yim JF, Sandinha T, Kerr JM, Ritchie D, Kemp EG. Treatment review of sight threatening circumscribed choroidal haemangioma. Int J Ophthalmol. 2010;3(2):168–71. https://doi.org/10.3980/j.issn.2222-3959.2010.02.18.

35. Cennamo G, Breve MA, Rossi C, Romano MR, de Crecchio G, Cennamo G. Transpupillary thermotherapy as a primary treatment for circumscribed choroidal haemangioma. Acta Ophthalmol. 2016;94(2):e167–9. https://doi.org/10.1111/aos.12810.

36. Gambrelle J, Kivela T, Grange JD. Sturge-Weber syndrome: decrease in intraocular pressure after transpupillary thermotherapy for diffuse choroidal haemangioma. Acta Ophthalmol. 2011;89(2):190–3. https://doi.org/10.1111/j.1755-3768.2009.01811.x.

37. Newman DK. Photodynamic therapy: current role in the treatment of chorioretinal conditions. Eye (Lond). 2016;30(2):202–10. https://doi.org/10.1038/eye.2015.251.

38. Schmidt-Erfurth UM, Michels S, Kusserow C, Jurklies B, Augustin AJ. Photodynamic therapy for symptomatic choroidal hemangioma: visual and anatomic results. Ophthalmology. 2002;109(12):2284–94.

39. Chan WM, Lim TH, Pece A, Silva R, Yoshimura N. Verteporfin PDT for non-standard indications—a review of current literature. Graefe's Arch Clin Exp Ophthalmol. 2010;248(5):613–26. https://doi.org/10.1007/s00417-010-1307-z.

40. Pilotto E, Urban F, Parrozzani R, Midena E. Standard versus bolus photodynamic therapy in circumscribed choroidal hemangioma: functional outcomes. Eur J Ophthalmol. 2011;21(4):452–8. https://doi.org/10.5301/ejo.2011.6263.

41. Su ZA, Tang XJ, Zhang LX, Su XH. Comparison of outcomes between overlapping-spot and single-spot photodynamic therapy for circumscribed choroidal hemangioma. Int J Ophthalmol. 2014;7(1):66–70. https://doi.org/10.3980/j.issn.2222-3959.2014.01.12.

42. Blasi MA, Tiberti AC, Scupola A, Balestrazzi A, Colangelo E, Valente P, Balestrazzi E. Photodynamic therapy with verteporfin for symptomatic circumscribed choroidal hemangioma: five-year outcomes. Ophthalmology. 2010;117(8):1630–7. https://doi.org/10.1016/j.ophtha.2009.12.033.

43. Hu Y, Chen Y, Chen L. Half-dosage and bolus injection photodynamic therapy for symptomatic circumscribed choroidal hemangioma: a case report. Photodiagn Photodyn Ther. 2015;12(3):526–9. https://doi.org/10.1016/j.pdpdt.2015.05.005.

44. Subira O, Brosa H, Lorenzo-Parra D, Arias-Barquet L, Catala-Mora J, Cobos E, Garcia-Bru P, Rubio-Caso MJ, Caminal-Mitjana JM. Choroidal haemangioma and photodynamic therapy. Anatomical and functional response of patients with choroidal hemangioma treated with photodynamic therapy. Arch Soc Esp Oftalmol. 2017;92(6):257–64. https://doi.org/10.1016/j.oftal.2016.11.013.

45. Huang S, Fabian J, Murray T, Shi W. Symptomatic circumscribed choroidal hemangioma undergoing PDT: VA outcomes. Optom Vis Sci. 2009;86(3):286–9. https://doi.org/10.1097/OPX.0b013e318196a724.

46. Xiong Y, Zhang F. Photodynamic therapy for circumscribed choroidal hemangioma. Zhonghua Yan Ke Za Zhi. 2007;43(12):1085–8.

47. Guagnini AP, De Potter P, Levecq L. Photodynamic therapy of circumscribed choroidal hemangiomas. J Fr Ophtalmol. 2006;29(9):1013–7.

48. Landau IM, Steen B, Seregard S. Photodynamic therapy for circumscribed choroidal haemangioma. Acta Ophthalmol Scand. 2002;80(5):531–6.

49. Hussain RN, Jmor F, Damato B, Heimann H. Verteporfin photodynamic therapy for the treatment of choroidal haemangioma associated with Sturge-Weber syndrome. Photodiagn Photodyn Ther. 2016;15:143–6. https://doi.org/10.1016/j.pdpdt.2016.06.009.

50. Nugent R, Lee L, Kwan A. Photodynamic therapy for diffuse choroidal hemangioma in a child with Sturge-Weber syndrome. J AAPOS. 2015;19(2):181–3. https://doi.org/10.1016/j.jaapos.2014.10.032.

51. Poh KW, Wai YZ, Rahmat J, Shunmugam M, Alagaratnam J, Ramasamy S. Treatment of diffuse choroidal haemangioma using photodynamic therapy. Int J Ophthalmol. 2017;10(3):488–90. https://doi.org/10.18240/ijo.2017.03.26.

52. Huiskamp EA, Muskens RP, Ballast A, Hooymans JM. Diffuse choroidal haemangioma in Sturge-Weber syndrome treated with photodynamic therapy under general anaesthesia. Graefe's Arch Clin Exp Ophthalmol. 2005;243(7):727–30. https://doi.org/10.1007/s00417-004-1102-9.

53. Cacciamani A, Scarinci F, Parravano M, Giorno P, Varano M. Choroidal thickness changes with photodynamic therapy for a diffuse choroidal hemangioma in Sturge-Weber syndrome. Int Ophthalmol. 2014;34(5):1131–5. https://doi.org/10.1007/s10792-014-9933-9.

54. Li KZ, Tan CS. Changes in choroidal thickness after photodynamic therapy for Sturge-Weber syndrome. Int Ophthalmol. 2015;35(5):615–6. https://doi.org/10.1007/s10792-015-0077-3.
55. Nagesha CK, Walinjkar JA, Khetan V. Choroidal neovascular membrane in a treated choroidal hemangioma. Indian J Ophthalmol. 2016;64(8):606–8. https://doi.org/10.4103/0301-4738.191512.
56. Mandal S, Naithani P, Venkatesh P, Garg S. Intravitreal bevacizumab (avastin) for circumscribed choroidal hemangioma. Indian J Ophthalmol. 2011;59(3):248–51. https://doi.org/10.4103/0301-4738.81051.
57. Sagong M, Lee J, Chang W. Application of intravitreal bevacizumab for circumscribed choroidal hemangioma. Korean J Ophthalmol: KJO. 2009;23(2):127–31. https://doi.org/10.3341/kjo.2009.23.2.127.
58. Anaya-Pava EJ, Saenz-Bocanegra CH, Flores-Trejo A, Castro-Santana NA. Diffuse choroidal hemangioma associated with exudative retinal detachment in a Sturge-Weber syndrome case: photodynamic therapy and intravitreous bevacizumab. Photodiagn Photodyn Ther. 2015;12(1):136–9. https://doi.org/10.1016/j.pdpdt.2014.12.002.
59. Chan LW, Hsieh YT. Photodynamic therapy for choroidal hemangioma unresponsive to ranibizumab. Optom Vis Sci. 2014;91(9):e226–9. https://doi.org/10.1097/opx.0000000000000349.
60. Querques G, Forte R, Querques L, Souied EH. Intravitreal ranibizumab for choroidal neovascularization associated with circumscribed choroidal haemangioma. Clin Exp Ophthalmol. 2011;39(9):916–8. https://doi.org/10.1111/j.1442-9071.2011.02580.x.
61. Bach A, Gold AS, Villegas VM, Wildner AC, Ehlies FJ, Murray TG. Spontaneous exudative retinal detachment in a patient with Sturge-Weber syndrome after taking arginine, a supplement for erectile dysfunction. Eye Vis. 2014;1:7. https://doi.org/10.1186/s40662-014-0007-x.
62. Paulus YM, Jain A, Moshfeghi DM. Resolution of persistent exudative retinal detachment in a case of Sturge-Weber syndrome with anti-VEGF administration. Ocul Immunol Inflamm. 2009;17(4):292–4. https://doi.org/10.1080/09273940902989357.
63. Sommers Smith SK, Smith DM. Beta blockade induces apoptosis in cultured capillary endothelial cells. In Vitro Cell Dev Biol Anim. 2002;38(5):298–304. https://doi.org/10.1290/1071-2690(2002)038<0298:bbiaic>2.0.co;2.
64. Giatromanolaki A, Arvanitidou V, Hatzimichael A, Simopoulos C, Sivridis E. The HIF-2alpha/VEGF pathway activation in cutaneous capillary haemangiomas. Pathology. 2005;37(2):149–51.
65. Sanz-Marco E, Gallego R, Diaz-Llopis M. Oral propranolol for circumscribed choroidal hemangioma. Case Rep Ophthalmol. 2011;2(1):84–90. https://doi.org/10.1159/000325142.
66. Leaute-Labreze C, Dumas de la Roque E, Hubiche T, Boralevi F, Thambo JB, Taieb A. Propranolol for severe hemangiomas of infancy. N Engl J Med. 2008;358(24):2649–51. https://doi.org/10.1056/NEJMc0708819.
67. Thapa R, Shields CL. Oral propranolol therapy for management of exudative retinal detachment from diffuse choroidal hemangioma in Sturge-Weber syndrome. Eur J Ophthalmol. 2013;23(6):922–4. https://doi.org/10.5301/ejo.5000322.
68. Bazin L, Gambrelle J. Combined treatment with photodynamic therapy and intravitreal dexamethasone implant (Ozurdex((R))) for circumscribed choroidal hemangioma. J Fr Ophtalmol. 2012;35(10):798–802. https://doi.org/10.1016/j.jfo.2012.06.015.
69. Quagliano F, Fontana L, Parente G, Tassinari G. Choroidal effusion after diode laser cyclophotocoagulation in Sturge-Weber syndrome. J AAPOS. 2008;12(5):526–7. https://doi.org/10.1016/j.jaapos.2008.03.014.
70. Lopez-Caballero C, Saornil MA, De Frutos J, Bianciotto C, Muinos Y, Almaraz A, Lopez-Lara F, Contreras I. High-dose iodine-125 episcleral brachytherapy for circumscribed choroidal haemangioma. Br J Ophthalmol. 2010;94(4):470–3. https://doi.org/10.1136/bjo.2009.160184.
71. Zografos L, Bercher L, Chamot L, Gailloud C, Raimondi S, Egger E. Cobalt-60 treatment of choroidal hemangiomas. Am J Ophthalmol. 1996;121(2):190–9.
72. Madreperla SA, Hungerford JL, Plowman PN, Laganowski HC, Gregory PT. Choroidal hemangiomas: visual and anatomic results of treatment by photocoagulation or radiation therapy. Ophthalmology. 1997;104(11):1773–8; discussion 1779.

73. Aizman A, Finger PT, Shabto U, Szechter A, Berson A. Palladium 103 (103Pd) plaque radiation therapy for circumscribed choroidal hemangioma with retinal detachment. Arch Ophthalmol. 2004;122(11):1652–6. https://doi.org/10.1001/archopht.122.11.1652.

74. Kubicka-Trzaska A, Karska-Basta I, Oleksy P, Romanowska-Dixon B. Management of diffuse choroidal hemangioma in Sturge-Weber syndrome with Ruthenium-106 plaque radiotherapy. Graefe's Arch Clin Exp Ophthalmol. 2015;253(11):2015–9. https://doi.org/10.1007/s00417-015-3061-8.

75. Frau E, Rumen F, Noel G, Delacroix S, Habrand JL, Offret H. Low-dose proton beam therapy for circumscribed choroidal hemangiomas. Arch Ophthalmol. 2004;122(10):1471–5. https://doi.org/10.1001/archopht.122.10.1471.

76. Levy-Gabriel C, Rouic LL, Plancher C, Dendale R, Delacroix S, Asselain B, Habrand JL, Desjardins L. Long-term results of low-dose proton beam therapy for circumscribed choroidal hemangiomas. Retina. 2009;29(2):170–5. https://doi.org/10.1097/IAE.0b013e31818bccfb.

77. Chan RV, Yonekawa Y, Lane AM, Skondra D, Munzenrider JE, Collier JM, Gragoudas ES, Kim IK. Proton beam irradiation using a light-field technique for the treatment of choroidal hemangiomas. Ophthalmologica. 2010;224(4):209–16. https://doi.org/10.1159/000260226.

78. Schilling H, Sauerwein W, Lommatzsch A, Friedrichs W, Brylak S, Bornfeld N, Wessing A. Long-term results after low dose ocular irradiation for choroidal haemangiomas. Br J Ophthalmol. 1997;81(4):267–73.

79. Ritland JS, Eide N, Tausjo J. External beam irradiation therapy for choroidal haemangiomas. Visual and anatomical results after a dose of 20 to 25 Gy. Acta Ophthalmol Scand. 2001;79(2):184–6.

80. Kim YT, Kang SW, Lee JI. Gamma knife radiosurgery for choroidal hemangioma. Int J Radiat Oncol Biol Phys. 2011;81(5):1399–404. https://doi.org/10.1016/j.ijrobp.2010.08.016.

81. Song WK, Byeon SH, Kim SS, Kwon OW, Lee SC. Gamma knife radiosurgery for choroidal haemangiomas with extensive exudative retinal detachment. Br J Ophthalmol. 2009;93(6):836–7. https://doi.org/10.1136/bjo.2008.151316.

82. Boixadera A, Garcia-Arumi J, Martinez-Castillo V, Encinas JL, Elizalde J, Blanco-Mateos G, Caminal J, Capeans C, Armada F, Navea A, Olea JL. Prospective clinical trial evaluating the efficacy of photodynamic therapy for symptomatic circumscribed choroidal hemangioma. Ophthalmology. 2009;116(1):100–105.e101. https://doi.org/10.1016/j.ophtha.2008.08.029.

83. Jurklies B, Anastassiou G, Ortmans S, Schuler A, Schilling H, Schmidt-Erfurth U, Bornfeld N. Photodynamic therapy using verteporfin in circumscribed choroidal haemangioma. Br J Ophthalmol. 2003;87(1):84–9.

84. Michels S, Michels R, Simader C, Schmidt-Erfurth U. Verteporfin therapy for choroidal hemangioma: a long-term follow-up. Retina. 2005;25(6):697–703.

85. Verbraak FD, Schlingemann RO, Keunen JE, de Smet MD. Longstanding symptomatic choroidal hemangioma managed with limited PDT as initial or salvage therapy. Graefe's Arch Clin Exp Ophthalmol. 2003;241(11):891–8. https://doi.org/10.1007/s00417-003-0765-y.

86. Singh AD, Kaiser PK, Sears JE, Gupta M, Rundle PA, Rennie IG. Photodynamic therapy of circumscribed choroidal haemangioma. Br J Ophthalmol. 2004;88(11):1414–8. https://doi.org/10.1136/bjo.2004.044396.

87. Porrini G, Giovannini A, Amato G, Ioni A, Pantanetti M. Photodynamic therapy of circumscribed choroidal hemangioma. Ophthalmology. 2003;110(4):674–80. https://doi.org/10.1016/s0161-6420(02)01968-1.

88. Dave T, Dave VP, Shah G, Pappuru RR. Diffuse choroidal hemangioma masquerading as central serous chorioretinopathy treated with oral propranolol. Retin Cases Brief Rep. 2016;10(1):11–4. https://doi.org/10.1097/icb.0000000000000165.

89. Kaushik S, Kaur S, Pandav SS, Gupta A. Intractable choroidal effusion with exudative retinal detachment in Sturge-Weber syndrome. JAMA Ophthalmol. 2014;132(9):1143–4. https://doi.org/10.1001/jamaophthalmol.2014.2464.